Evidence-based Research Methods for Chinese Medicine

Siu-wai Leung · Hao Hu
Editors

Evidence-based Research Methods for Chinese Medicine

Springer

Editors
Siu-wai Leung
Institute of Chinese Medical Sciences
University of Macau
Macau
China

Hao Hu
Institute of Chinese Medical Sciences
University of Macau
Macau
China

ISBN 978-981-10-9583-2 ISBN 978-981-10-2290-6 (eBook)
DOI 10.1007/978-981-10-2290-6

Softcover reprint of the hardcover 1st edition 2016

Printed on acid-free paper

This Springer imprint is published by Springer Nature
The registered company is Springer Science+Business Media Singapore Pte Ltd.

Preface

Chinese medicine, in spite of its long history in development of theories and practices, has been questioned by scientists in terms of modern scientific methods. It would be understandable that traditional Chinese medicine was developed well before modern sciences and cannot have full specification, standardized records, and rigorous statistical design and analysis of experiments all at once. While not all modalities of Chinese medicine have fully developed appropriate scientific methods, some Chinese medicine research methods have been standardized with proper definitions to acquire, analyze and evaluate research results, making Chinese medicine more evidence-based/led. We believe that the evidence-based/led Chinese medicine research will unlock the potentials and demonstrate the effectiveness of Chinese medicine to become a crucial part of health systems. To this end, we organized a series of workshops on Good Research and Scientific Publishing (GRASP) and invited some of the workshop lecturers to write about their current methods and tools for Chinese medicine research.

This series of workshops was co-organized by the Institute of Chinese Medical Sciences (ICMS) at the University of Macau and the International Society for Chinese Medicine (ISCM) in Macao. ISCM is an independent and not-for-profit academic organization mainly funded by the Macao Foundation. ISCM has been maintaining an international platform to promote modernization and internationalization of Chinese medicine. In particular, ISCM is running the Chinese Medicine journal published by BioMed Central (BMC) to promote evidence-led Chinese medicine.

Chinese Medicine journal is an open-access, peer-review academic journal, which has been indexed by the Science Citation Index Expanded (SCI-E) since July 2013, with a journal impact factor of 1.58 according to the 2015 Journal Citation Reports (JCR). It also follows the international publication guidelines, including Committee on Publication Ethics (COPE), BMC and Springer Nature's guidelines, to promote good research practices among Chinese medicine researchers. The journal currently publishes three types of articles, i.e., evidence-based/led, scientifically justified, and ethical research reports (research articles), systematic literature reviews (review articles) and commentaries on evidence-based/led research (commentary articles).

The mission to advocate the evidence-based/led Chinese medicine as well as ethical journal editorial process inspired us to organize the GRASP workshops. From the workshops, we noticed so many exciting methodological innovations that would be helpful to meet the methodological challenges in Chinese medicine research. All of these motivated us to take a further step to compile this small collection ("toolbox") of current methods for those who are eager to start or advance their evidence-based/led research in Chinese medicine. We look forward to further innovations and practical publications on rigorous research methods from and for the Chinese medicine community.

Macau, China
2016

Siu-wai Leung
Hao Hu

Acknowledgments

We are indebted to many researchers contributed to the GRASP workshops and this book, especially the chapter reviewers:

Name	Institution
Jing Cai	University of Macau
Hui-juan Cao	Beijing University of Chinese Medicine
Arthur de Sá Ferreira	Augusto Motta University
Xinfeng Guo	Guangzhou University of Chinese Medicine
Wenxue Hong	Yanshan University
Simon Ming-Yuen Lee	University of Macau
Peng Li	University of California
Liming Lu	Guangzhou University of Chinese Medicine
Luigina Mortari	Universita degli Studi di Verona
Josiah Poon	The University of Sydney
Zehuai Wen	Guangzhou University of Chinese Medicine
Elena Wilson	La Trobe University

We would like to express our sincere thanks to Dr. Daniel Chi-Wai Tse, the President of the International Society for Chinese Medicine (ISCM). As a founder of ISCM, Dr. Tse conceived the ideas of "evidence-led Chinese medicine" and initiated the Chinese Medicine journal. He is our role model. We also thank Prof. Yitao Wang, the General Secretary of ISCM and the Director of Institute of Chinese Medical Sciences (ICMS) at the University of Macau, for his kind support for our work.

We thank all GRASP workshop participants, invited lecturers, and student helpers for running the workshops. We also thank Cadmon Sze Chung Yuen for his administrative support and chapter proofreading. Last but not the least, we are grateful to our funding agencies, the Macao Foundation and the University of Macau, for supporting the workshop.

Contents

Contributors

Terje Alraek Institute of Health Sciences, Kristiania University College, Oslo, Norway; Department of Community Medicine, Faculty of Health Sciences, National Research Center in Complementary and Alternative Medicine (NAFKAM), UiT The Arctic University of Norway, Tromsø, Norway

Stephen Birch Institute of Health Sciences, Kristiania University College, Oslo, Norway

Cui-Zan Cai State Key Laboratory of Quality Research in Chinese Medicine, Institute of Chinese Medical Sciences, University of Macau, Macau, China

Hui-juan Cao Centre for Evidence-Based Chinese Medicine, Beijing University of Chinese Medicine, Beijing, China

Hong Chen State Key Laboratory of Quality Research in Chinese Medicine, Institute of Chinese Medical Sciences, University of Macau, Macau, China

Xin Chen State Key Laboratory of Quality Research in Chinese Medicine, Institute of Chinese Medical Sciences, University of Macau, Macau, China

Yuanyuan Cheng School of Chinese Medicine, University of Hong Kong, Hong Kong, China

Arthur Sá Ferreira Laboratory of Computational Simulation and Modeling in Rehabilitation, Augusto Motta University Center, Rio de Janeiro, RJ, Brazil

Xinfeng Guo Key Unit of Methodology in Clinical Research, Guangdong Provincial Hospital of Chinese Medicine, Guangzhou University of Chinese Medicine, Guangzhou, China

Jiang He State Key Laboratory of Quality Research in Chinese Medicine, Institute of Chinese Medical Sciences, University of Macau, Macau, China

Zhen-dan He Department of Pharmacy, School of Medicine, Shenzhen University, Shenzhen, China

Hao Hu State Key Laboratory of Quality Research in Chinese Medicine, Institute of Chinese Medical Sciences, University of Macau, Macau, China

Kun Hyung Kim Department of Acupuncture and Moxibustion, Korean Medicine Hospital, Pusan National University, Yangsan, Korea

Myeong Soo Lee Clinical Research Division, Korea Institute of Oriental Medicine, Daejeon, Korea

Siu-wai Leung State Key Laboratory of Quality Research in Chinese Medicine, Institute of Chinese Medical Sciences, University of Macau, Macau, China

Jian Li Faculty of Arts and Humanities, University of Macau, Macau, China

Min Li School of Chinese Medicine, Hong Kong Baptist University, Hong Kong, China

Jian-ping Liu Centre for Evidence-Based Chinese Medicine, Beijing University of Chinese Medicine, Beijing, China

Yat-Tung Lo State Key Laboratory of Phytochemistry and Plant Resources in West China (CUHK), LDS YYC R&D Centre for Chinese Medicine, School of Life Sciences, The Chinese University of Hong Kong, Hong Kong, China

Jia-Hong Lu State Key Laboratory of Quality Research in Chinese Medicine, Institute of Chinese Medical Sciences, University of Macau, Macau, China

Liming Lu Key Unit of Methodology in Clinical Research, Guangdong Provincial Hospital of Chinese Medicine, Guangzhou University of Chinese Medicine, Guangzhou, China

Ingrid Jardim Azeredo Souza Oliveira Laboratory of Computational Simulation and Modeling in Rehabilitation, Augusto Motta University Center, Rio de Janeiro, RJ, Brazil

Jianhui Rong School of Chinese Medicine, University of Hong Kong, Hong Kong, China

Pang-Chui Shaw State Key Laboratory of Phytochemistry and Plant Resources in West China (CUHK), LDS YYC R&D Centre for Chinese Medicine, School of Life Sciences, The Chinese University of Hong Kong, Hong Kong, China

Hutcha Sriplung Epidemiology Unit, Faculty of Medicine, Prince of Songkla University, Songkhla, Thailand

Zehuai Wen Key Unit of Methodology in Clinical Research, Guangdong Provincial Hospital of Chinese Medicine, Guangzhou University of Chinese Medicine, Guangzhou, China

Ka-Lok Wong State Key Laboratory of Phytochemistry and Plant Resources in West China (CUHK), LDS YYC R&D Centre for Chinese Medicine, School of Life Sciences, The Chinese University of Hong Kong, Hong Kong, China

Ming-Yue Wu State Key Laboratory of Quality Research in Chinese Medicine, Institute of Chinese Medical Sciences, University of Macau, Macau, China

Xuesong Yang Dermatology Department, Yunnan Provincial Hospital of Traditional Chinese Medicine, Kunming, China

Sze Chung Yuen State Key Laboratory of Quality Research in Chinese Medicine, Institute of Chinese Medical Sciences, University of Macau, Macau, China

Jia Zhao School of Chinese Medicine, University of Hong Kong, Hong Kong, China

Chapter 1
Introduction

Sze Chung Yuen, Hao Hu and Siu-wai Leung

Abstract Chinese medicine (CM) has been questioned for more than a century about its inadequate scientific evidence. While some past CM studies were not convincing from the views of modern sciences, especially under critical appraisal by evidence-based medicine (EBM), we hold a positive view that CM can demonstrate its effectiveness in improving healthcare through the same evidence-based, or even a more extensive evidence-led, approach. In the last decade, standardized CM research methods have been enabling researchers to acquire, analyze, and evaluate evidence scientifically. This book is a practical guide to the latest methods, including design and conduct of CM research according to applicable EBM guidelines. The authors of all chapters in this book are active CM researchers in their fields of research, including clinical studies, informatics, laboratory studies, pharmaceutical administration, pharmacy research practices, research ethics, and socio-medical studies. Many chapters also cover the best practices of research ethics and scientific reporting in their fields. We anticipate that Chinese medicine would bring the valuable knowledge to current healthcare by following these EBM research methods.

Keywords Chinese medicine (CM) · Methodology · International standards and guidelines · Evidence-based medicine · Evidence-led medicine

S.C. Yuen (✉) · H. Hu · S. Leung
State Key Laboratory of Quality Research in Chinese Medicine, Institute of Chinese Medical Sciences, University of Macau, Macau, China
e-mail: syue0101@gmail.com

H. Hu
e-mail: haohu@umac.mo

S. Leung
e-mail: swleung@umac.mo

S. Leung and H. Hu (eds.), *Evidence-based Research Methods for Chinese Medicine*, DOI 10.1007/978-981-10-2290-6_1

1.1 Objectives

This book provides a practical guide to the evidence-based medicine (EBM) research methods, including their design and execution that are suitable for Chinese medicine (CM). Through these research methods, we would like to introduce the international standards and guidelines of EBM applicable to Chinese medicine research, particularly good research practices (GRP), medical research ethics and scientific reporting.

1.2 Clinical Research

1.2.1 Chapter 2 Methodology for Clinical Studies Investigating Chinese Medicine

CM is usually regarded as a modality of complementary medicines that are lacking scientific evidence for their efficacy to participate into the mainstream health systems. This chapter described the methodology used to measure the clinical efficacy of CM using randomized controlled trials (RCT), observational studies and meta-analytic studies. The authors emphasized the importance of (a) experimental controls (placebos or active controls) to demonstrate the efficacy, (b) randomization to avoid biases in sampling and group allocation, (c) proper sample size calculation to avoid invalid statistical inference, (d) blinding to avoid performance bias and detection bias, and (e) ethical practices to avoid research misconduct. To ensure the quality of clinical trials, we must clearly define the objectives in terms of PICOS (i.e., patients, intervention, comparison, outcomes and study design) at the first place. The study protocol submitted to the ethics committee for ethics approval should include the full study design and executable procedures of the trial. The protocol must be registered with one of the public trial registries, e.g., Australian New Zealand Clinical Trials Registry and Chinese Clinical Trial Registry. The authors described the execution of RCTs in terms of study management, data management, data analysis, report writing and publication. Besides RCTs, they also discussed the merit and weakness of observational studies, e.g., case studies, case series, cross-sectional studies, case-control studies, and cohort studies. The meta-analytic studies, e.g., systematic reviews, and meta-analyses, measure the clinical efficacy of CM by aggregating the results of evidence-based research. For each type of these studies, the authors provided an example to illustrate the key concepts.

1.2.2 Chapter 3 Effectiveness Assessment of Chinese Medicine in Clinical Research

For evaluating clinical effectiveness, RCT is usually regarded as the best scientific method (i.e., gold standard). The method can avoid common biases, e.g., selection bias and detection bias by random allocation of participants, statistical calculation of sample sizes, blinding in out-come assessment, and clear definition of eligibility criteria of participants. In practice, there are common issues of RCTs for evaluating the clinical effectiveness of CM. It is a challenge to use placebos in the control group; e.g. the color, odor, taste, and smell of CM decoction may not be easily mimicked. Universal outcome indicators for many diseases in CM treatment are unavailable; thus, selecting appropriate indicators would not be easy for CM research. The authors took chronic obstructive pulmonary disease (COPD) as an example to demonstrate why few RCTs can use appropriate indicators. In addition to the selection of indicators, the authors also discussed the issues in patient-reported outcome analysis, safety assessment and health economics evaluation. These different evaluation purposes differentiates the trial into (a) the efficacy trials that measure the expected results under experimental conditions, and (b) the effectiveness trials that measure the beneficial effects. These different trials may use different outcome measures. Unlike Western medicine (WM), the clinical effectiveness of CM should be measured according to the *zheng* (syndrome)-oriented model of CM, although the measures of many syndromes in CM are still subjective and lacking well-recognized definitions in *zheng* (syndrome) differentiation. This chapter exemplified how to evaluate the effectiveness of combined CM and conventional psychotherapy in treating menopausal syndrome.

1.2.3 Chapter 4 Placebo Controlled Trials in Acupuncture: Problems and Solutions

Acupuncture procedure involves the stimulation of acupoints, mainly through needles. Inserting needles to specific acupoints to accurate depths by correct manipulation techniques is believed to trigger certain sensations, particularly "*deqi*", in human subjects. Due to inadequate controls and acupuncture techniques, both positive and negative efficacy findings of acupuncture were obtained from clinical trials. In particular, when the sham acupuncture (e.g., shallow needle insertion with no manipulation, sage-dagger like needle without skin penetration) was used as control, the small differences between treatments and controls raised questions about the efficacy of acupuncture. This chapter focused on how to address the current issues of using sham acupuncture in RCTs. Among different types of sham acupuncture being used in RCTs, some techniques, e.g., sham TENS and sham laser, would not be suitable for use as controls since human subjects can easily identify the needling methods. The authors conducted a systematic review on the use of sham acupuncture and real acupoints to determine whether there are clinical effects of sham acupuncture per se. The systematic review showed that sham acupuncture as controls was often more effective than, or sometimes as effective as, the real acupuncture treatment. The authors found no inert sham acupuncture, even when shallow penetration or nonpenetration was used. They suggested that the effects of sham acupuncture in RCTs should be interpreted with care as we do not fully understand the underlying mechanism of acupuncture.

1.3 Healthcare Data Acquisition and Analysis

1.3.1 Chapter 5 Qualitative Interview for Chinese Medicine Research: Challenges and Prospects

The preferences of CM over WM in Chinese population were attributed to the sociomedical factors such as lifestyles, social cultures, and educational backgrounds. Such healthcare preferences can be related to consumer preferences for particular CM products. Qualitative interview is an useful approach to exploring about "how" and "why" of such socio-medical phenomena. A proper interview allows participants to express their views accurately, efficiently, and informatively. This chapter explained how to apply qualitative interview in CM research. The authors described the major procedures of qualitative interview, including the design and execution of interview protocols, sampling schemes, and data analysis. Instead of random sampling from a big population, qualitative interview often uses nonrandom sampling to target a specific population. Such nonrandomized sampling approach would require researchers to specify detailed criteria for selecting the potential participants in the protocol according to the research objectives, which must be clearly defined in advance. For specific purposes, different approaches (e.g., thematic and comparative approaches) and styles (e.g., structured, semi-structured, and in-depth interviews) are applicable. The thematic approach aims to identify not only the key themes but also their inter-relationships. The comparative approach aims to overcome the cultural biases in sampling, interview questions, and conceptual communication. To overcome the communication barrier, the authors suggested that some WM practices can be used to explain to the interviewees who are not familiar with the CM terms. Before conduct of any part of an interview (e.g., participant recruitment), its full protocol must be approved by an ethics committee. To illustrate the main issues of qualitative interview, the authors took a previous study as an example for interviewing consumers at community pharmacies for their attitudes towards and opinions about Chinese patent medicine and Western chemical drugs.

1.3.2 Chapter 6 A Need for Standard Data Collection Procedures in Studies on Traditional Chinese Medicine

In CM, the clinical diagnosis are highly dependent on CM practitioners' subjective judgment in *zheng* (syndrome) differentiation. WM had used similar subjective observations to identify most diseases until late nineteenth century. Such disease diagnosis based on subjective observations as a methodological paradigm was then shifted to that based on more objective measurements. Compared to the WM of the present day, CM is much like the judgment-laden (or even theory-laden) psychiatry in clinical diagnosis. This chapter described an application of the Delphi technique to standardize a data collection method for *zheng* differentiation. Through expert group communication with multiple iterations in the Delphi technique, the experts can reach consensus and decide specific items to be in a standardized checklist for data collection. In this chapter, the authors reviewed the procedures of the Delphi technique applicable to (a) item selection to record all disease-related signs and symptoms, (b) formulation of a checklist according to the expert consensus, and (c) publication and implementation of the clinical diagnosis method. There should have a steering committee of senior experts who can select an expert panel and inform them of the study objectives and provide substantial feedback. The process should be iterated for multiple rounds to formulate a consensual checklist. The checklist may employ semi-quantitative scales instead of the quantitative ones to measure the severity degrees and confidence of clinical observations so that the practitioners can reason about the actual such uncertainties. The observation should be extensive and the data should include the temporal variability of clinical signs or *zheng*. To group related clinical signs and symptoms into a *zheng*, the authors suggested proper statistical methods such as latent class analysis and cluster analysis.

1.3.3 Chapter 7 Methods for Assessment of Interrater Reliability for Diagnosis and Intervention in Traditional Chinese Medicine Studies

While clinical information can be systematically collected through checklist-based methods, *zheng* differentiation could be still biased among different raters. The raters' agreement in clinical diagnosis would help increase confidence in the results of *zheng* differentiation. Studies on inter-rater agreement in *zheng* differentiation are much needed to ensure the accuracy of CM clinical diagnosis. This chapter reviewed the assessment methods of rater reliability and diagnostic accuracy in *zheng* differentiation. The authors provided useful information about compliance with ethical issues, requirements for sample size calculation, recruitment of participants, selection criteria for raters, design of questionnaire, and statistical analysis of the collected data. To test the *zheng* differentiation algorithm, the authors used SimTCM for *zheng* simulation to generate manifestation profiles. They also advised that the simulation should be based on a database with the *zheng* of interest. The sample sizes of both participants and multiple (e.g., five) raters should be statistically determined. The raters' judgment on each simulated participant should be tabulated for statistical analysis. Accuracy, sensitivity, specificity, and predictive values are common diagnostic performance indicators. The authors recommended to use κ statistic for univariate cases and ι coefficient for multivariate cases.

1.3.4 Chapter 8 Bioinformatics for Molecular Authentication of Chinese Medicinal Materials

The quality and efficacy of CM herbal formula would be impossible to assure without correct identification of CM herbs. The morphology of herbs is not necessarily adequate to authenticate herbal species. DNA barcoding is a more reliable authentication method. A DNA barcode is a short sequence (or its pattern) with high inter-specific variability and low intra-specific variability in the genomic region flanked by conserved regions that would facilitate primer design. For herbal authentication by DNA barcoding, bioinformatics help identify and compare numerous samples of DNA sequences. This chapter focused on DNA sequencing and DNA fingerprinting. For DNA sequencing, the authors described the procedures for extraction, amplification, and sequencing of DNA samples for identifying the barcodes, followed by bioinformatics analysis for comparing the unknown sequences in the samples with the available reference (known) sequences in the major DNA databases, including NCBI, Flora of China, IPNI, Tropicos, ING, MPNS, BOLD and MMDBD. Three common DNA sequence formats, i.e., FASTA, ASN.1, and XML, were used in accordance their compatible platforms or software. Sequence alignment softwares were used, e.g., BLAST programs for local alignment and Clustal programs for global alignment, to estimate the similarities and distances among sequences. For region-specific fingerprinting, the authors recommended to use SCAR and PCR-RFLP to reduce DNA degradation and achieve higher reproducibility. The authors also warned that many DNA sequences from databases have not been thoroughly verified; thus, the sequence data should be used with caution.

1.4 Laboratory Research

1.4.1 *Chapter 9 Proteomic Response Fingerprinting (ProReF) for Rapid Identification of Protein Targets for Chinese Medicine*

A CM treatment usually covers multiple drug targets and biological pathways; however, it is difficult for conventional experimentation to simultaneously investigate those multiple drug targets and their underlying action mechanisms. This complexity hindered our research for understanding of the molecular pharmacology behind the scene. This chapter introduced an omics approach, namely proteomic response fingerprinting (ProReF), to simultaneously investigate large scale expression, modification and interaction of proteins in cells and tissues for the biological responses to CM treatment. ProReF consists of two main parts, two-dimensional gel electrophoresis for cellular protein separation based on the isoelectric points and molecular weights of proteins, and mass spectrometry (MS) for protein identification. The comparison of the ProReF results from different treatments and controls will help identify the specific biological responses to specific CM treatments. Besides the working principle, the authors detailed the experimental procedures, including sample preparation, protein separation by two-dimensional gel electrophoresis, protein imaging and comparison, spot extraction, trypsin digestion of proteins, peptide identification by MS and bioinformatics analysis, and experimental verification and mechanistic studies by Western blotting. Many useful techniques were suggested for each critical step, e.g., the protein spots with upregulated expression should be selected from the CM-treated gel, while the protein spots with downregulated expression should be selected from the control gel. The authors took a previous ProReF study as an example to demonstrate how amygdalin did significantly alter expression of 11 proteins. The authors summarized other applications of ProReF to CM research into cancer, inflammation, neurological diseases and diabetes, e.g., how the protein targets of amygdalin from *Semen Persicae* and puerarin from Radix *puerariae lobatae* were identified. They also advised new researchers about crucial tips to carry out successful protein identification, especially the sensitivity of protein detection, the use of databases for protein identification, and the functional annotation of proteins.

1.4.2 *Chapter 10 Chinese Medicine in Neurological Diseases: Pharmacological Perspective*

Several CM herbal formula (e.g., *Huanglian Jiedu Decoction*), single herbs [e.g., *Pueraria Montana* var. *lobata* (Willd) (*Gegen*)], and herbal extracts [e.g., berberine from *Coptis chinensis* Franch (*Huanglian*)] are commonly used to treat neurological diseases. This chapter focused on the CM treatments for stroke, Parkinson's disease (PD) and Alzheimer's disease (AD) and the animal disease models used to study these neurological diseases. For AD, transgenic animal models are available. For stroke, four-vessel occlusion model and two-vessel model are applicable. The pathophysiological and pharmacological effects on stroke being studied include inflammatory pathways, cell apoptosis, and platelet aggregation, oxidative stress, glutamate-induced excitatory toxicity, and extracellular GABA dysfunction. The effects on AD cover inflammation, oxidative stress, apoptosis, and Aβ accumulation, induction of autophagy, and regulation of APP process. For PD, the effects include apoptosis, oxidative stress, protein aggregation, neural immune and inflammatory responses, mitochondrial energy metabolism, and induction of autophagy. The pathophysiology and CM pharmacogenomics of these diseases were also related to genomic variations.

1.4.3 Chapter 11 Effects of Chinese Medicinal Components of Chemokine Receptors: Theory, Results and Methodology

Chemokine receptors are involved in various immune functions, e.g., inflammation and infection. Chemokines possess highly specific activities, e.g., inducing cell migration without activation. Chemokine receptor antagonists block chemokines binding to their receptors, consequently inhibit the chemotactic effects and generate specific therapeutic effects. Due to the relatively specific effects with only limited side effects, chemokines become potential drug targets in many disease treatments. This chapter reviewed the recent development of chemokine receptor antagonists (e.g., experimental protocols used to discover chemokine receptor antagonists from CM) and their clinical trials. The development of chemokine receptor antagonists was often challenging due to low plasma drug levels, off-target effects, and inactivity in human body. The authors exemplified the development of chemokine receptor antagonists from CM with three examples including shikonin, bile acid, and tannic acid. These three compounds blocked the chemotaxis by inhibition of the chemokine receptor expression and functions, blockade of fMLP receptors, and inhibition of SDF-1α/CSCR4 interactions, respectively. Three experimental methods, i.e., chemotaxis assay, calcium mobilization, and binding assay, were described. Chemotaxis assay uses a filter to form two compartments, i.e., lower compartment loaded with chemokines and upper compartment filled with cell suspension, for monitoring the changes in leukocyte mobilization to either compartment after CM treatment. Elevation and mobilization of cytosolic calcium in response to chemokines binding can be monitored by using calcium chelators as fluorescent calcium dyes. The binding of CM to chemokine receptors is experimentally verifiable after incubating the cell line transfected with chemoattractant receptor with radiolabeled chemokine ligands in the presence of CM. The scientific significances, working principles, procedures and, techniques of the development of chemokine receptor antagonists introduced in this chapter should be helpful to young researchers in this field.

1.5 Concluding Remarks

For innovative applications of scientific methods to advance CM, the authors presented the best EBM methods to their knowledge. They are also aware that these methods still have limitations to overcome in the future. We hope that these methods can be complemented with one another to inspire their users to conduct new research into evidence-based CM.

Chapter 2
Methodology for Clinical Study Investigating Chinese Medicine

Hui-juan Cao and Jian-ping Liu

Abstract *Background* A new clinical trial guideline for Chinese Medicine (CM) was published in 2015, which incorporates the characteristics of traditional approaches of practice with the practical recommendations of rigorous research methodology. *Objectives* This chapter aimed to introduce the research methodology for CM practice and the key considerations that need to address in relation to the characteristics of CM as a whole system. *Details* This chapter includes the introduction of basic study design, key issues on planning, implementing, and analyzing and reporting a clinical study of CM. The principles of clinical study design, basic research methods for interventional studies (e.g., randomized controlled trial), observational studies (e.g. cohort study, case-control study, case series study and case report), and systematic reviews were introduced in the first section. For each type of study, research model, scope of application, merit and weakness were addressed in accordance with the characteristics of CM. In the second section, we introduce details of methods of planning (research question, study protocol, sample size, study settings, participants, comparisons, and outcome measures), implementing (allocation sequence generation, blinding method, ethical approval, bias control, data management and monitoring), and analyzing (statistical methods, analysis and interpretation of results) a CM clinical study. Adequate examples from previous publications are shown to give clues and deepen understanding on each issue. *Conclusions* It is our hope that this chapter will encourage a thoughtful and meticulous process of investigation to provide reliable evidence for CM therapies for better health care.

Keywords Study methodology · Chinese medicine

H. Cao (✉) · J. Liu
Centre for Evidence-Based Chinese Medicine, Beijing University of Chinese Medicine, Beijing, China
e-mail: huijuancao327@hotmail.com

J. Liu
e-mail: jianping_l@hotmail.com

S. Leung and H. Hu (eds.), *Evidence-based Research Methods for Chinese Medicine*, DOI 10.1007/978-981-10-2290-6_2

2.1 Introduction to Basic Study Design

2.1.1 Principles of Clinical Study Design

2.1.1.1 Control

Regarding the natural course of disease, spontaneous fluctuations and regression to mean phenomenon, the results of a study are hard to interpret without a strict control. "Control" means that a sample of participants with consistent diagnosis and baseline characteristics are divided into several groups receiving different kinds of treatment, to demonstrate the differences in the results between the experimental and control groups. The group of patients who receive nonexperimental treatment is usually called control group. The overall finding is that a study without an appropriate control is more likely to report positive results of the treatment. With a control group(s), we could compare the outcomes of the experimental and control groups and find the difference between them to determine the treatment effect.

Commonly used "control group" include blank control (no treatment for this group), placebo (ineffectual treatment) control, standard (effective treatment with evidence) control, mutual control (a comparison of two different doses or different routes of administration for treatment), self control (participants may accept two therapies one after another), paired control (subjects of the experimental group are matched with the control group according to the non-test factors), and historical control (to compare the current patients with previous patients who had received standard treatment) [1]. For different purpose of research, we may choose different type of comparisons (Table 2.1). Among them, placebo control is unlikely to be successful in trial assessing traditional Chinese medicine (TCM) due to the absence of ideal placebo for most of the Chinese medicine therapies, especially the non-pharmaceutical treatment such as acupuncture, cupping therapy, etc. We may further discuss this in the sections below.

Table 2.1 Potential type of controls for different research purpose

Type of effect assessed	Comparisons	Type of controls
Effect beyond natural history	A versus blank	Blank control
Specific effect (efficacy)	A versus placebo	Placebo control
Nonspecific effect (effectiveness)	A plus B versus B	Standard control (B)
Comparative effect	A versus C	Mutual control, or other nonstandard control (C)

2.1.1.2 Equalization

Equalization aims to make sure the comparability of characteristics of participants between groups, and besides matching and stratifying, the most popular method to fulfill equalization is randomization. Randomization, whenever during sampling from general population or allocating samples into different groups, is a method to ensure each individual of the sample/population has equal opportunity to be selected/divided to the treatment or control group. The purposes of randomization are (a) to avoid selection bias caused by choosing patients with preference; and (b) to meet the basic requirements of statistical analysis such as significance tests.

Although historically "manual" randomization techniques (such as throwing dice, flipping coin, and drawing straws) were used, statistical software (such as SPSS and SAS) are now commonly used to generate the random numbers [2].

2.1.1.3 Replication

Replication may test the internal and external validity of the study. There are two implications: one is to reproduce the study results under the same test condition; the other is to observe appropriate sample size of participants within the study. The reproducibility of the results indicates that it is not caused by chance. And the stable result seems more reliable.

On the other hand, in clinical trials it is crucial to be able to differentiate a chance from a true effect. Statistical methods should be used to determine the sample size of the study.

2.1.1.4 Blinding

In any clinical study, if neither the patient himself, practitioner nor outcome assessor is aware of which treatment the patient is receiving, it is called a blinding study. Physicians may pay more attention to the patients in placebo group and enhancing the placebo effect; participants may seek to other treatments when they were allocated to control group; outcome assessors may check the data of treatment group carefully to detect bias. The purpose of "blinding" is to avoid the performance bias, detection bias, or reporting bias due to subjective factors.

Blinding would be feasible if the following aspects are met: (a) ethics, the double-blind procedure as well as the application of placebo control should not result in any harm or undue risk to a patient; (b) practicality, as we mentioned before, for some non-pharmaceutical Chinese medicine treatment (such as acupuncture, cupping therapy, moxibustion, qigong, etc) it would be infeasible to arrange a double-blind trial due to the lack of ideal placebo control as well as patient previous experience of the treatment; (c) avoidance of bias, researchers need to assess just how serious the bias might be without blinding; and (d) compromise, in some cases only partial blinding (e.g., independent blinded evaluators) would be sufficient to minimize the potential bias [3].

2.1.1.5 Ethics

For every clinical study, ethics issue should be concerned throughout the design and conduct period according to the Declaration of Helsinki issued by the World Medical Association in 1964 and revised in 2013. Depending on the content of the study, getting approval from the ethics committee (or IRB, institutional review board) can be challenging and time consuming. The following documents should be prepared at the beginning of the study to get approval from ethics committee.

1. Study protocol
2. Written informed consent form
3. Patient information leaflet
4. Case report form (CRF) during the study
5. Patient recruitment procedures, including advertisements
6. Safety information for intervention treatment, including drugs or nondrug treatment
7. Investigators' current curriculum vitae and/or other documentation providing evidence of qualifications and competence.

2.1.2 Basic Research Methods for Observational Studies

Descriptive studies and analytic studies are the two types of observational studies. Descriptive studies describe distribution characteristics of disease in relation to variables such as person, place, and time. The data provided by descriptive studies are essential for public health administrators as well as epidemiologists. The ultimate goal of an analytic study is to determine a particular exposure causes or developing preventive procedures for the specific disease. Common descriptive studies are case reports, case series studies, and cross-sectional studies; and frequently used analytic studies are case-control studies and cohort studies.

2.1.2.1 Case Reports/Case Series Studies

A single case study is an observational study of an individual patient who exposes to certain interventions which produced meaningful results. A case report usually

Table 2.2 Results of uncontrolled observational studies

	Outcomes		Total
	+	−	
Exposure/intervention	*a*	*b*	$a + b$

concerns about clinical diagnosis, demographic characteristics, details of treatment, prognosis, and follow-up of the case. The purpose of the study is to explore the potential relationship between specific intervention and outcomes through the individual's detailed medical information or records. However, due to the large variation of an individual person, the results of a case report may only provide weak evidence of clinical experience for the clinicians. Usually, case reports can represent and document the first clues in the identification of a new disease or the adverse effects of exposures in unusual medical occurrences. Key points on designing a single case study include (a) developing the protocol according to research purpose; (b) calculating a sample size; (c) identifying appropriate patient through strict diagnostic, inclusion and exclusion criteria; (d) collecting data precisely and completely; and (e) evaluating the outcomes objectively and independently by all the researchers.

The results of a case series are collected from a number of individual cases, which may occur within a fairly short period of time. The collection of a case series can mean the difference between formulating a useful hypothesis and merely documenting an interesting medical oddity (Table 2.2).

Merits of case reports and case series studies:

1. This design can be used for the studies in which control is unavailable due to ethics issue;
2. This kind of studies can be used to observe the patients who do not meet the inclusion criteria of clinical controlled trials, and provide the potential evidence for those patients;
3. This kind of studies can be used to observe a special disease (tumor, AIDS, atypical pneumonia, etc.), rare or chronic disease, complications and adverse reactions; and
4. This kind of studies cost less and is easy to carry out.

Demerits of case reports and case series studies:

1. While case reports and case series are very good for generating hypotheses, they are not applicable to verifying hypotheses;
2. Their external validity is not determined; and
3. These two types of studies are usually considered to have many potential confounding factors, and more likely to overestimate the effect under observation.

Example 2.1 [4]
Introduction: To evaluate the therapeutic effect of traditional medicinal cupping for treatment of fibromyalgia.

Methods: A prospective case series was conducted in 30 consecutive patients with fibromyalgia at an outpatient department in a hospital in Beijing. Patients were diagnosed according to the criteria of 1990 by American College of Rheumatology. The bamboo cup, boiled in herbal decoction for 5 min, was applied to Ashi (tender) points for 10 min once daily for 15 sessions. Visual analog scale (VAS, 0–10 cm) for pain and the number of tender points were recorded at the baseline, 5, 10, 15 days, and followed up at 2 weeks after the treatment.

Results: The average score of VAS in 30 patients was 2.63 sessions. Visual analog scale (VAS, 0–10 cm) for pain and the number of tender points were recorded at the baseline, 5, 10, 15 days, and followed up at 2 weeks after t29 of Rheumatology. The bamboo cup, tender points was reduced from 12.57 ± 2.25 at 5 days, 11.2 ± 2.50 at 10 days, to 9.33 ± 2.89 at 15 days. Compared with baseline, VAS score was reduced 52.27 %, and the number of tender points was reduced 30.86 %. 29 patients were followed up to 2 weeks and the VAS and tender points sustained (1.24 ± 0.67 for VAS; 9.07 ± 2.96 for pain points). There was no serious adverse effect occurred during the treatment.

Conclusions: Medicinal cupping therapy appears to relieve pain in patients with fibromyalgia in terms of VAS and number of tender points, and the promising effect deserves to be tested in clinical trials.

2.1.2.2 Cross-Sectional Studies

Cross-sectional studies, also called surveys, usually provide information about the frequency and characteristics of a disease by furnishing a snapshot of the health experience of the population at a specified time. Within a survey, potential exposure and disease/health status are assessed simultaneously among individuals in a well-defined population. The results from cross-sectional studies can help public health administrators to assess the health status and healthcare needs of a population. On the other hand, cross-sectional studies can also be used to provide information on the prevalence of disease or other health outcomes in certain occupations.

There are two key points of cross-sectional study: (a) Exposure and disease status are assessed at a single point in time, it is impossible to determine whether the exposure is the cause of the disease or an outcome of the development of the disease; and (b) Since prevalence rather than incidence must be considered in cross-sectional study, the data obtained will always reflect determinants of survival as well as etiology.

Merits of cross-sectional studies:

1. A cross-sectional study is population-based study, which may have strong external validity;
2. The concurrent control is formed naturally during the survey, therefore, the comparability between groups is stronger;
3. A variety of factors can be observed at the same time.

Demerits of cross-sectional studies:

4. Disease and factors exist at the same time, it is difficult to refer the causal relationship;
5. Incidence rate cannot be calculated in cross-sectional study;
6. Latent period and remission patients are easy to be misdiagnosed; and
7. It is generally applicable to the study of chronic disease.

Only in one case, a cross-sectional study can be considered as a special type of analytic study and used to test hypotheses. This can occur only when the current values of the exposure variables are unmodifiable over time, thus representing the value present at the beginning of the disease. However, in most cross-sectional study, the exposures may be subject to alteration subsequent (or even consequent) to the development of disease. Under these circumstances, the data can be used to describe characteristics of individuals with the disease and to formulate hypotheses, but not to validate them.

Example 2.2 [5]

Background: The prevalence of chronic kidney disease is high in developing countries. However, no national survey of chronic kidney disease has been done incorporating both estimated glomerular filtration rate (eGFR) and albuminuria in a developing country with the economic diversity of China. We aimed to measure the prevalence of chronic kidney disease in China with such a survey.

Methods: We did a cross-sectional survey of a nationally representative sample of Chinese adults. Chronic kidney disease was defined as eGFR less than 60 mL/min per 1.73 m^2 or the presence of albuminuria. Participants completed a lifestyle and medical history questionnaire and had their blood pressure measured, and blood and urine samples taken. Serum creatinine was measured and used to estimate glomerular filtration rate. Urinary albumin and creatinine were tested to assess albuminuria. The crude and adjusted prevalence of indicators of kidney damage were calculated and factors associated with the presence of chronic kidney disease analyzed by logistic regression.

Findings: 50,550 people were invited to participate, of whom 47,204 agreed. The adjusted prevalence of eGFR less than 60 mL/min per 173 m^2 was 1.7 % (95 % CI 1.5–1.9) and of albuminuria was 9.4 % (8.9–10.0). The overall prevalence of chronic kidney disease was 10.8 % (10.2–11.3); therefore the number of patients with chronic kidney disease in China is estimated to be about 119.5 million (112.9–125.0 million). In rural areas, economic development was independently associated with the presence of albuminuria. The prevalence of chronic kidney disease was high in north (16.9 % [15.1–18.7]) and southwest (18.3 % [16.4–20.4]) regions compared with other regions. Other factors independently associated with kidney damage were age, sex, hypertension, diabetes, history of cardiovascular disease, hyperuricaemia, area of residence, and economic status.

Interpretation: Chronic kidney disease has become an important public health problem in China. Special attention should be paid to residents in economically improving rural areas and specific geographical regions in China.

2.1.2.3 Case-Control Studies

A case-control study is a retrospective study, in which subjects are selected on the basis of whether they do (cases) or do not (controls) have a particular disease/outcome under study. Its basic principle is to compare the proportion having a history of an exposure or characteristic of interest between the cases and controls to evaluate the association between the exposure and a disease/outcome. This type of study design is more commonly used in the early exploration of the relationship between disease and its possible etiological factors.

For a case-control study to verify the association between an exposure and disease, comparability of cases and controls is essential (Table 2.3). The aspects of comparability that must be considered include factors such as their baseline risk of developing the disease other than from the exposure under study, as well as the accuracy and completeness of data. Consequently, the major issues to be considered in designing and conducting a case-control study are the selection of the study groups and the sources of information about exposure and disease.

Table 2.3 Results of case-control studies

		Outcomes		Total
		+	–	
Exposure/interventions	Yes	a	b	$a + b$
	No	c	d	$c + d$
Total		$a + c$	$b + d$	$a + b + c + d$

Example 2.3 [6]

Ethnopharmacological relevance: Our previous study indicated that the TCM formula Liu-Wei-Di-Huang-Wan, which consists of six types of herbs, namely Rehmannia glutinosa (Gaertn.) DC., root, dried; Cornus officinalis Siebold & Zucc., fructus, dried; Dioscorea oppositifolia L., root, dried; Alisma plantago-aquatica subsp. orientale (Sam.) Sam., tuber, dried; Paeonia × suffruticosa Andrews, bark, dried; Poria cocos (Fr.) Wolf., sclerotium, dried, is the most frequently prescribed herbal formula used to treat type 2 diabetes patients. The aim of the study was to evaluate the integration of TCM into diabetes care in terms of how it reduces the risk of developing kidney failure.

Materials and methods: The Taiwan's National Health Insurance Research Database (NHIRD) provided detailed information of healthcare services for each patient and covers 98 % of all Taiwan residents as of 2007. Case and control subjects were selected from the NHIRD. Two multivariable logistic regression models were constructed in order to explore two types of exposure assessments including prescription of TCMs (model 1) and prescription of different estimated dosages of Liu-Wei-Di-Huang-Wan (model 2).

Results: Using logistic regression model 1, having used TCMs was independently associated with a decreased risk of kidney failure by multivariable analysis (OR = 0.69, 95 % CI 0.61–0.77). Using logistic regression model 2, there was no difference between non-Liu-Wei-Di-Huang-Wan TCM users and Liu-Wei-Di-Huang-Wan TCM users in terms of the risk of developing kidney failure. Furthermore, there was also no linear dose-response trend when we used exposure to prescribed Liu-Wei-Di-Huang-Wan as a continuous variable (for non-Liu-Wei-Di-Huang-Wan TCM users, OR = 0.68, 95 % CI 0.60–0.77; for TCM users consuming 1–30 g of Liu-Wei-Di-Huang-Wan, OR = 0.69, 95 % CI 0.54–0.87; for >30 g of Liu-Wei-Di-Huang-Wan, OR = 0.84, 95 % CI 0.49–1.44).

Conclusions: Integrating TCM health care into diabetes care was found to be associated with a decreased risk of developing kidney failure. Having recognized the use of TCM, exploring any potential interactions and adverse effects, and integrating both technologies into a holistic treatment system may be beneficial to the relief of diabetic nephropathy on patients with type 2 diabetes.

Merits of case-control studies:

1. As a retrospective study, outcome measurement of this kind of studies is easy to meet the ethical requirements;
2. With a small sample size, it is commonly used for etiology research of rare disease and the special long latency disease;
3. By asking the history of the exposure, most of the research are short-term study which saves manpower and material resources and easy to draw conclusions; and

4. Case-control study is able to explore a variety of potential etiologic exposures that might relate to the specific disease as well as the internal connections among these factors.

Demerits of case-control studies:

1. It is insufficient for the evaluation of rare exposures, unless the attributable risk is high, and in some situations, it is difficult to establish the temporal relationship between exposure and disease;
2. Selection bias can occur whenever the inclusion of cases or controls into the study depends in some way on the exposure of interest, which is a problem in case-control study;
3. Recall bias, which related to differences in the ways exposure information is recalled or reported by cases and what truly happened, exist in every case-control study and should be considered carefully in the design as well as in the interpretation of published results;
4. Observation bias, or information bias in gathering information from participants, may also be a particular problem in a case-control design; and
5. Cannot directly compute morbidity rate of disease in both groups, unless the study is population based.

2.1.2.4 Cohort Studies

In a cohort study, the observed individuals are grouped by whether or not they are exposed to a certain kind of suspected risk factor for a disease. Cohort studies have great advantages for evaluating the association between risk factors and disease. (a) participants exposure are determined when the disease has not yet occurred, thus, the time sequence of the exposure and disease can be more clearly established; (b) this type of study is more suitable for assessing effects of rare exposures, especially those arise in occupational settings; and (c) cohort studies allow for the test of multiple effects of a single exposure.

Cohort studies are generally classified into prospective or retrospective cohort studies or two-way cohort studies. In retrospective cohort studies, both exposures and outcomes of interest have already occurred when the study is initiated. In prospective studies, the diseases have certainly not yet occurred, regardless whether or not the relevant exposures have occurred at the time when the study begun. Consequently, participants must be followed into the future to assess incidence rates of disease after the selection of the cohort (Table 2.4). Ambidirectional cohort study

Table 2.4 Results of cohort studies

Exposure/interventions	Outcomes		Total
	+	−	
Yes	a	b	$a + b$
No	c	d	$c + d$
Total	$a + c$	$b + d$	$a + b + c + d$

is mixed of the prospective and retrospective studies, which is usually most useful for exposures having both short-term and long-term effects.

Merits of cohort studies:

1. Cohort studies can test multiple effects of a single exposure;
2. For etiology study, the incidence or mortality of the exposed group and control group can be obtained directly, and the cause of the disease can be directly analyzed; and
3. The prospective cohort study which minimizes bias in the ascertainment of exposure, can interpret temporal relationship between exposure and disease.

Demertis of cohort studies:

1. Cohort studies are insufficient for the evaluation of rare diseases, unless the attributable risk is high;
2. Prospective cohort study can be extremely costly, while retrospective cohort study requires the sufficient records; and
3. Validity of the results can be seriously affected by missing data.

Example 2.4 [7]

Background: Chinese medicine is commonly used and covered by health insurance to treat symptoms of uterine fibroids in Taiwan. This retrospective cohort study compared the consumption of conventional western medicine and medical cost between CM users and nonusers among patients with uterine fibroids.

Methods: We extracted 44,122 patients diagnosed with uterine fibrosis between 1996 and 2010 from the National Health Insurance reimbursement database, which is a population-based database released by a government-run health insurance system. Multivariate linear regression models were used to find association between using CM and the consumption of conventional medicine, and between using CM and medical cost.

Results: The total fibroid-related conventional western medicine consumed by CM users was less than that by nonusers ($\beta = -10.49$, $p < 0.0001$). Three categories of conventional medicines, including antianemics (−3.50 days/year/patient, $p < 0.0001$), hemostatics (−1.89 days/year/patient, $p < 0.0001$), and hormone-related agents (−3.13 days/year/patient, $p < 0.0001$), were used less in patients who were CM users. Moreover, although using CM increased 16.9 USD per patient in CM users annually ($p < 0.0001$), the total annual medical cost for treating fibroid was 5610 USD less in CM users than in nonusers ($p < 0.0001$).

Conclusions: Our results suggested that CM reduced the consumption of conventional medicine, and might be a potential therapeutic substitute for conventional western medicines to treat uterine fibroids with low cost.

Table 2.5 Results of randomized controlled trials

	Outcomes		Total
	+	−	
Intervention	a	b	$a + b$
Control	c	d	$c + d$
Total	$a + c$	$b + d$	$a + b + c + d$

2.1.3 Basic Research Methods for Intervention Studies

Intervention studies, or clinical trials, are generally considered either therapeutic or preventive. The therapeutic trials are conducted on the patients with a particular disease to determine the ability of a therapy to eliminate symptoms, prevent recurrence, or reduce mortality from that disease. The preventive trials are to assess whether a procedure avoids the occurrence of disease among those free from that condition at enrollment.

2.1.3.1 Randomized Controlled Trials

Randomized controlled trials (RCT) are commonly used to evaluate the effects of medical interventions, health education or management. Since random allocation is the basis of designing RCT, which means the eligible participants would be randomly allocated to the experimental group or control group, cause–effect relationship could be evaluated according to the results from RCT due to the comparability between baseline characteristics of two groups and well-controlled confounding factors during the treatment. Consequently, RCT is generally accepted as the golden standard study model for assessing therapeutic effects of specific drugs/procedures.

In a randomized controlled trial, participants, regardless of random sampling or not, must be identified through accepted diagnostic criteria and met the inclusion and exclusion criteria of the study. They would then be randomly assigned to the experimental or control group to receive corresponding treatments. Outcomes are measured before, during, and after the treatment. According to the types of data, appropriate statistical methods would be used to analyze the reliably observed effect of the intervention and the differences between groups (Table 2.5).

Example 2.5 [8]

Background: Perennial allergic rhinitis (PAR) has a high and increasing prevalence worldwide. Ear acupressure (EAP) is a noninvasive semi-self-administered form of acupuncture. Previous studies indicated that EAP could be effective and safe for AR symptom management. However, there was insufficient evidence to confirm this. This study investigated whether EAP, a noninvasive clinical alternative to acupuncture, is effective and safe for PAR.

Methods: This is an international, multicenter, randomized, single-blind, sham-controlled trial. The trial was conducted at two centers: Royal Melbourne Institute of Technology University (Melbourne, Australia) Clinical Trial Clinic and Guangdong Provincial Hospital of Chinese Medicine, Guangzhou, China. PAR participants were randomized to receive real or sham EAP treatment once a week for 8 weeks and then were followed up for 12 weeks. Participants were instructed to administer EAP stimulation three times daily. Symptom severity and quality of life (QoL) were evaluated. Adverse events (AEs) were also monitored. Intention-to-treat analysis on change of symptom scores and QoL was applied.

Results: Two hundred forty-five participants were randomly assigned to real (n = 124) and sham EAP (n = 121) groups. Twenty-five participants discontinued during treatment and 15 participants dropped out during follow-up. At the end of treatment and follow-up periods, changes of global QoL score were significantly greater in the real EAP group compared with the sham group. At the end of follow-up, scores for total nasal symptom, runny nose, and eye symptoms in the real EAP group had a greater reduction compared with the sham group. Overall, both real and sham EAP were well tolerated. Two severe AEs were reported but were not considered related to the EAP procedures.

Conclusions: In conclusion, EAP showed short-term and extended benefit for improving PAR symptoms and QoL for PAR patients.

Merits of randomized controlled trials:

1. If the treatments are allocated at random in a representative sample of sufficiently large size, RCT has the potential to provide a degree of assurance about the validity of a result that is simply not possible with any observational study; and
2. Results of RCT can provide the strongest and most direct epidemiologic evidence that the basis of whether an observed association is a causal judgment.

Demerits of randomized controlled trials:

1. RCT cost more than most observational studies;
2. Ethical considerations hold back the assessment of many treatments or procedures in RCT; and
3. There is a more strict inclusion criterion for those who participate in RCT compare to other observational studies or pragmatic studies, the external validity is therefore comparatively limited.

According to the purpose of the study, there are several types of randomized controlled trials including explanatory RCT (which tests efficacy in a research setting with highly selected participants and under highly controlled conditions), pragmatic RCT (which design is closer to the "real world" clinical circumstances and conditions), crossover trial (a type of longitudinal study in which subjects receive a sequence of different interventions), N-of-1 trial (which is considered as a crossover randomized controlled trial with only one subject), dose-response study (which is a valid research design to determine the best dose of the intervention product), factorial design (which allows researchers to assess more than one intervention in a single trial), etc. Among those different types of RCTs, explanatory RCT is commonly used to evaluate the efficacy of the intervention (drugs), ideally there should be reasonable placebo control for the intervention. Pragmatic RCT is more often to focus on the comparison of the effectiveness between different interventions, thus it can be classified into the category of comparative effectiveness research (see Sect. 2.1.4).

2.1.3.2 Nonrandomized Controlled Trials

A well-designed nonrandomized comparative study may have higher external validity compared to randomized trial, and the recruitment of that kind of study is much easier than for randomized trial due to patients' strong preference. What we need to concern when designing nonrandomized trial are taking baseline differences into account, and adjusting analyses for imbalances.

Example 2.6 [9]
Background: One of five children visiting a homoeopathic physician is suffering from atopic eczema.

Objective: To examine the effectiveness, safety, and costs of homoeopathic versus conventional treatment in usual care.

Methods: In a prospective multicentre comparative observational nonrandomized study, 135 children (homoeopathy $n = 48$ vs. conventional $n = 87$) with mild to moderate atopic eczema were included. The primary outcome was the SCORAD (Scoring Atopic Dermatitis) at 6 months. Further outcomes at 6 and 12 months also included quality of life of parents and children, use of conventional medicine, treatment safety and disease-related costs.

Results: The adjusted SCORAD showed no significant differences between the groups at both 6 months (homoeopathy 22.49 ± 3.02 [mean $\pm$ SE] vs. conventional 18.20 ± 2.31, $p = 0.290$) and 12 months (17.41 ± 3.01 vs. 17.29 ± 2.31, $p = 0.974$). Adjusted costs were higher in the homoeopathic than in the conventional group: for the first 6 months EUR 935.02 versus EUR 514.44, $p = 0.026$, and for 12 months EUR 1524.23 versus EUR 721.21, $p = 0.001$. Quality of life was not significantly different between both groups.

Conclusions: Taking patient preferences into account, homoeopathic treatment was not superior to conventional treatment for children with mild to moderate atopic eczema.

In some cases, randomization may not be appropriate even if the control group is available. First, the patients who visit TCM or integrative medicine hospital seeking to Chinese medicine therapies usually prefer to Chinese medicine treatments. This may increase the difficulty of recruiting appropriate patients for a randomized controlled trial. Also, randomization is not necessary to find out whether treatment effects are very different if the study is well done in other respects. Moreover, randomization is also not appropriate for the comparison of anthroposophical and conventional care if we are primarily interested in the differences regarding preferences, experiences, processes, and compliance.

2.1.4 Basic Research Methods for Comparative Effectiveness Research

Efficacy is the specific effects which are due to the active ingredient of the treatment, while effectiveness is both of the specific and nonspecific effects, latter are those due to psychological or psycho-physiological effects associated with the act of treatment (such as placebo effect). Placebo control and appropriate blinding methods are needed to investigate the efficacy of the components; otherwise, the specific effect could not be validated. However, challenges exist when conducting RCTs for traditional nondrug therapies (e.g. acupuncture, cupping therapy, and moxibustion). Therapeutic effects can be influenced by patient preference, practitioner preference, and patient–practitioner relationship, among others, rather than the efficacy of the interventions themselves. Thus, placebo control could be extremely difficult for nondrug therapies, specific study design such as comparative effectiveness research (CER) could be used to investigate the effectiveness of such therapies [10].

CER, which is defined as "conduct and synthesis of systematic research comparing different interventions and strategies to prevent, diagnose, treat, and monitor health conditions," is aimed to assist patients, practitioners, purchasers, and policy makers to make informed decisions which may improve health care at both the individual and population levels. Design models of CER could be like majority of the observational studies, some of the experimental studies (especially pragmatic randomized controlled trials) and research synthesis (such as systematic review, see Sect. 2.1.5). Observational studies are more likely to be chosen to evaluate the effectiveness of the interventions since their implementation conditions are closer to the environment of the real world.

On the other hand, the primary and secondary outcomes of the CER are more concerned with the patient-centered outcomes, which are selected as the core of the patients' interests [11]. Consequently, CER is also called 'patient-centered outcome research'.

2.1.5 Basic Research Methods for Systematic Review and Meta-analysis

Different from the above original studies, systematic review is a kind of secondary study. Systematic review, defined as a kind of study which acquire, appraise, and synthesis evidence from scientific studies in order to provide informative, empirical answers to the research questions, is considered the 'gold standard' for assessing the effectiveness of a treatment or intervention. In another word, systematic review brings together all available research evidence with critical appraisal of the quality of the studies. This information can then be combined with your clinical judgment to make decisions about how to deliver the best care to your patients.

Meta-analysis [12], which also called quantitative systematic review, looks at data from multiple studies of the same clinical question and uses a variety of statistical techniques to integrate their findings. A systematic review may or may not have meta-analysis within it, if a systematic review did not conduct meta-analysis due to the potential heterogeneity among included studies, it would be called qualitative or descriptive systematic review.

The Cochrane collaboration is an independent, nonprofit, nongovernmental organization consisting of a group of more than 31,000 volunteers in more than 120 countries, which conducts systematic reviews of mainly randomized controlled trials of healthcare interventions and published them in the Cochrane Library. The Cochrane Handbook [13] outlines eight general steps for preparing a systematic review:

1. Defining the question and formulating the inclusion and exclusion criteria;
2. Literature searching;
3. Screening and selecting studies, then extracting data;
4. Assessing methodological qualities of included studies;
5. Analyzing and pooling the data;
6. Addressing reporting biases;
7. Presenting results and "summary of findings" tables; and
8. Interpreting results and drawing conclusions.

Merits of systematic review:

1. Systematic review could identify the heterogeneity among studies and merge those trials with acceptable homogeneity;
2. Minimize or eliminate the bias of included studies and achieve the currently 'best evidence';
3. Weakness of systematic review;
4. Grade of evidence of systematic review is depending on the quality of original studies included; and
5. Misuse of systematic review or meta-analysis may overestimate the effect of interventions or controls.

Example 2.7 [14]

Objective: Cupping as a traditional therapy is used to treat a myriad of health conditions, including pain. This systematic review assessed the effectiveness and safety of cupping for different types of pain.

Methods: Thirteen databases and four trial registries were searched for randomized clinical trials. Meta-analysis of data was conducted if there was nonsignificant clinical and statistical heterogeneity (measured by I^2 test) among trials.

Results: Sixteen trials with 921 participants were eligible and included. Six trials were assessed as low risk of bias, another six trials were of unclear risk of bias, and the remaining four trials were of high risk of bias. Pain was related to three acute and seven chronic diseases. Meta-analysis showed a beneficial effect of cupping compared to wait-list control (visual analogue scale (VAS), MD 1.85 cm, 95 % CI 2.66–1.04) and heat therapy (numerical rating scale, MD 2.05 cm, 95 % CI 2.93–1.17). Cupping combined with acupuncture was superior to acupuncture alone on posttreatment pain intensity (VAS, MD 1.18 cm, 95 % CI 1.68–0.68), however, no difference was found between this comparison based on changes in pain intensity (difference of VAS, MD 0.16 cm, 95 % CI 0.54–0.87). Results from other single studies showed significant benefit of cupping compared with conventional drugs or usual care. Hematoma and pain at the treated site, increasing local pain or tingling were reported as mild adverse effects of cupping.

Conclusion: This review suggests a potential positive short-term effect of cupping therapy on reducing pain intensity compared with no treatment, heat therapy, usual care, or conventional drugs.

Currently, hundreds of the CM systematic reviews are published annually. However, findings from 70 Cochrane reviews [15] related to herbal medicine and acupuncture showed insufficient evidence to support or to refute the intervention due to either poor methodology quality or small sample size of the included trials. It is important to direct future research by two ways based on the Cochrane review conclusions, one is to address how to shape the research questions in relation to traditional CM (see Sect. 2.2.1.1), and the other is how to design clinical trials to raise the quality.

2.2 Key Issues in Planning, Implementing, Analyzing, and Reporting a Clinical Study

2.2.1 Planning

2.2.1.1 Defining a Research Question

Raising a research question is the first and important part of whole research program. A clear research question is the precondition for deciding which choice of design makes sense, which patients should be included, which interventions and controls should be discussed and which outcomes should be measured. That is the reason why posing the research question appropriately is absolutely fundamental.

After translating clinical problems into questions (no matter background question or foreground question), these questions should be further structured as PICO (S):

1. P: patients, or what kind of population would be concerned in the research;
2. I: intervention, or exposure you interest;
3. C: comparison;
4. O: outcomes that would be primary or secondary measured and reported in the research; and
5. S: study type, which would be determined according to the study purpose.

Once the research question is formulated, you should search online (at least through PubMed, http://www.ncbi.nlm.nih.gov/pubmed or CNKI, cnki.net) to find out whether the similar studies have already been conducted or ongoing. You may further revise or redefine your research question according to the current evidence. During this process, the specific research objectives would be confirmed.

2.2.1.2 Drafting the Study Protocol

Study protocol is a document that describes the objectives, type of research model, methodology, statistical methods, and procedures of a clinical study. Developing the study protocol is a process that goes hand in hand with planning the study. The protocol describes the whole study in detail before the study started.

One should probably draft the study protocol cover the following items:

1. Study objectives and background

In this section, researchers should state the rational of the study clearly, including the importance of subject area, review of relevant literature, study justification, relevant research questions and how will the research results be used.

2. Research team

Principle investigator (PI) is the person responsible for the implementation and quality control of clinical trial, who must be qualified to ensure the quality of clinical trial. Research team would be constituted by persons whose expertise in methodology, statistics, clinical study and the relevant majors.

3. Overview of research design

To clarify what kind of study model it may employ, and describe the details of the study design. For observational studies, methods of selecting participants, defining exposure, measuring outcomes, and analyzing data should be fully addressed. And for intervention studies, methods of randomization and blinding are quite important in the protocol.

4. The inclusion criteria, exclusion criteria of the participants

Researchers should describe the characteristics of participants and disease clearly, study setting, as well as the procedures of recruitment, advertising plan, and recruitment materials.

If the aim of the study is to determine a specific effect of intervention, using adequate placebo control is required, and to ensure blinding and to minimize bias the placebo should be indistinguishable from the study intervention. As mentioned before, there was no ideal placebo control for most of the TCM therapies. In fact, placebos could be easily used in drug trial, if placebo and drugs have indistinguishable in appearance, smell, and taste. Therefore, for herbal medicine, capsules could be an option. For nondrug Chinese medicine therapies, sham acupuncture is the contention. Neither standard needles inserted at inappropriate sites nor non-penetrating needles were impure placebo. And for cupping therapy, massage, tai chi, or other type of meditation therapy, placebo control seems difficult to simulate. For assessing those kinds of interventions, comparative effectiveness research could be considered.

5. Sample size estimation

Total number and number in each group, including all assumptions as recalculation might be necessary. To determine the size of a study, researchers should consider the main purpose of the study, type of primary outcome measures, methods of statistics, and potential difference of effect between groups.

6. Details of the intervention and control

Details of intervention and control should be thorough enough to make sure that other researchers could repeat the study step by step according to your protocol.

7. Clinical observation and outcome measures

All patients should be regularly followed up, and examined at a certain interval of time. Time of each observation and inspection should be clearly reported in the protocol, and if available, in the case report form (CRF) as well. Primary and secondary outcomes should be outlined.

8. Design of case report form

The CRF is used to record the data in clinical trials, in which how patient response to the drug along with their general information should be noted. At meanwhile, the baseline condition of the patients should also be recorded.

9. Adverse events and severe adverse events
10. Data management and statistical analysis

Data management includes establishing the database, inspection and verification the data, and statistical analysis. In the protocol, plan of statistical analysis should be mentioned, such as the basic statistical methods, types of hypothesis (superiority, equivalence or non-inferiority test) etc.

11. Quality control of clinical trials

It is advisable at a very early stage to plan how to handle trial results as they materialize. Monitoring the trial is to ensure the clinical trials conducted following the predefined way and get the accurate records/data. Methods of monitoring should be stated clearly in the protocol.

12. Publishing the research

The belonging of the research findings (including the publications) should be clarified in the protocol.

Example 2.8 [16]
Background: Conducting randomized controlled trials on traditional Chinese nondrug therapies has been limited by factors such as patient preference to specific treatment modality. The aim of this study is to investigate the feasibility of applying a partially randomized patient preference (PRPP) trial model in evaluating the efficacy of two types of TCM therapies, acupuncture and cupping, for fibromyalgia while accounting for patients' preference of either therapeutic modality.

Methods: This protocol was approved by the Institutional Ethics Committee of affiliated Dongfang Hospital, Beijing University of Chinese Medicine (approval number: 2013052104-2). One hundred participants with fibromyalgia will be included in this study. Diagnosis of fibromyalgia will be based on the American College of Rheumatology criteria. Before treatment, participants will be interviewed for their preference toward acupuncture or cupping therapy. Fifty participants with no preference will be randomly assigned to one of the two groups and another 50 participants with strong preference to either acupuncture or cupping will receive what they choose. For acupuncture and cupping therapy, the main acupoints used will be tender points (Ashi). Treatment will be three times a week for 5 consecutive weeks with a follow-up period of 12 weeks. Outcome measures will be qualitative (patient expectation and satisfaction) and quantitative (pain intensity, quality of life, depression assessment).

Trial registration number: NCT01869712 (in clinicaltrials.gov, on 22nd May 2013).

2.2.1.3 Registering the study

After getting an approval from the Ethics Committee, and before starting recruitment, we suggest that the researchers should register the study online. International Medical Journal editorial board requires all clinical trials to be internationally registered before publishing, regarding to ethical aspect (Table 2.6). The readers or other researchers are allowed to check the study plan and make their own decisions

Table 2.6 List of trial registries

Name of registries	Abbreviations	Country	Website	Date established
Australian New Zealand Clinical Trials Registry	ANZCTR	Australia/New Zealand	http://www.anzctr.org.au/	2003
Brazilian Clinical Trials Registry	REBEC	Brazil	http://www.ensaiosclinicos.gov.br/	2010
Chinese Clinical Trial Registry	Chi-CTR	China	http://www.chictr.org/cn/	2005
Clinical Research Information Service	CRIS	Korea	http://cris.nih.go.kr/cris/en/	2009
Clinical trials.gov	–	USA	http://clinicaltrials.gov/	1997
Clinical Trials Registry-India	CTRI	India	http://www.ctri.in/	2007
Cuban Public Registry of Clinical Trials	RPCEC	Cuba	http://registroclinico.sld.cu/	2009
EU Clinical Trials Register	EU-CTR	Europe	https://www.clinicaltrialsregister.eu/	2004
German Clinical Trials Register	DRKS	Germany	https://drks-neu.uniklinik-freiburg.de/drks_web/	2008
International Standard Randomized Controlled Trial Number Register	ISRCTN	UK	http://www.controlled-trials.com/	2003
Iranian Registry of Clinical Trials	IRCT	Iran	http://www.irct.ir/	2008
Japan Primary Registries Network	JPRN	Japan	http://rctportal.niph.go.jp/	2002
Pan African Clinical Trial Registry	PACTR	Africa	http://www.pactr.org/	2008
The Netherlands National Trial Register	NTR	Netherlands	http://www.trialregister.nl/	2004
Sri Lanka Clinical Trials Registry	SLCTR	Sri Lanka	http://www.slctr.lk/	2008

on the methodological quality of the study. According to a study [17] which investigated the inconsistent between registered protocol and final report of the study, particularly inconsistent reporting of primary outcomes is a major violation of trial design for confirmatory studies. This may introduce a potential high risk of reporting bias, and downgrade the internal validity and evidence of the study results.

When the investigators register their trials with the above registries, they should provide the following information: study title, program code, funding resources, study type, settings, diagnostic/inclusion/exclusion criteria for participants, details of intervention and control, outcome measurements, timing of the study and contact information.

2.2.2 *Implementing*

2.2.2.1 Study Management

Study management is process containing plans, it organizes and manages to allow successful completion of specific project objectives. Initiation, planning, execution, monitoring/controlling, and completion are all need to be managed in a clinical study. Challenges of study management include: (a) to achieve all of these objectives within the limits of the known constraints of the project such as scope, time and budget; and (b) to optimize the allocation of resources to meet the objectives as efficiently as possible.

Commonly more months are spent running a trial than planning it or analyzing its data. A schedule with certain timelines of the study would be really helpful to control the study process. Besides, finances, roles, and functions in study team, monitoring (as we mentioned in 'drafting study protocol' section) are also important on managing study. Sometimes, taking notes (using checklist or mind mapping) in a structured way is helpful.

2.2.2.2 Data Management

All data should be collected, double checked, and organized before analysis. The appropriate forms for each patient should be arranged and distributed to each investigator at the beginning of the trial. It should be clarified who is responsible for completing each form. The handling of clinical trial data at the coordinating center requires administrative and clerical skills which should not be the priority of clinicians or statisticians. In addition, a specially trained data manager whose job is to get all trial data in good shape ready for statistical analysis is needed. For most cases, a data monitoring committee (DMC) will also be required by local standards.

For each form arriving at the coordinating center, the DMC should carry out a series of checks:

1. General checks, to make sure that all forms have been sent at the right time and received with matched patient number;
2. Missing data;
3. Range checks, to ensure that no items fall within the in appropriate range of replies; and
4. Logical checks, to find out any inconsistencies in replies to different questions.

Any problems identified by these checks should be conveyed back to the local institution so that corrections can be made. Data managers will also have concerns with the subsequent data processing which often requires use of computer software (such as EpiData).

2.2.3 *Analyzing*

2.2.3.1 Steps of Data Analysis

With a specific research question and clarified protocol, we could predefine a statistical analysis plan (SAP) of the study, and this actually should be more detailed than the relevant part of protocol.

1. To analyze the data, you should first define the analysis populations and the handling of missing values. If no data are present for the variable in the current time point, appropriate statistical methods (such as last value carried forward or multiple imputations for a continuous variable, and the worst/best case scenario for a categorical variable) should be used to deal with missing data.
2. Then, people should choose suitable statistical methods, which depend on the variable types and sample size. Statistical methods may include methods for descriptive analysis, confirmatory analysis and multiple testing.
3. The next step is performing the statistical analysis. The researchers may need to use statistical software and become fully conversant with the software. Do not forget to check the data and the results for plausibility and recalculate the important results. Any document of the statistical analysis including notes, USB sticks, or mobile hard drives should be clearly labeled and safely stored for at least five years after termination of the study.
4. The last key step is to interpret the results and draw conclusions. Remember that the conclusions should be clearly based on your study question and should consider the potential limitations of the study.

2.2.3.2 Basic Principles of Statistical Analysis

For each patient in a clinical trial one collects three types of data: (a) which treatment the patient assigned to and actually received; (b) the patients response to the treatment including adverse events; and (c) details of the patient's initial condition and previous history before entry into the trial.

When describing the data, one should describe the basic three types of response data in clinical trials, which are qualitative response, quantitative response, and time to relapse. Frequencies or constitution ratios could be reported as qualitative response, and it is essential to record the total number of patients on each treatment; otherwise, one cannot reliably interpret the results. For quantitative data, the simplest summary is to compute the mean response with the confidence interval for the patients on each treatment. Thus, one can check if the values are clinically feasible and valid to reduce the possibility of erroneous extreme results.

Significant tests have become the most commonly used methods of statistical inference in clinical trials, and both statistical and clinical significance should be assessed and interpreted.

2.2.4 Reporting

Through publication, research findings can be spread worldwide. Researchers who are concerned with a similar topic may repeat the study or test its conclusions. On the other hand, the publication may help others to avoid wasting time and resources to do redundant work. It may provide the current 'best evidence' for some specific interventions and help clinicians to make decisions.

2.2.4.1 Early Preparation for Publication

One should decide on a number of basic issues as early as possible.

1. Defining the aims;
2. Deciding on authorship;
3. Selecting a journal;
4. Checking instructions for authors; and
5. Checking general guidelines for reporting.

When selecting the journal, researchers may consider the field of research topics, impact factors (which reflect the impact of the journal), and the quality of the journal (such as its PubMed list or peer review system). Each journal may have its own instructions for authors. Different journals may have different ways to list author names, format the abstract, or cite references. That is the reason why people should read the instructions and find out which format the journal prefers before drafting.

2.2.4.2 Writing the Manuscript

Reports of original clinical research and systematic reviews are usually structured: introduction/background (why did you start), objectives (what's the main purpose), methods (what did you do), results (what did you find), discussions (what does it mean), and conclusions (what you finally concluded).

High-ranking journals often require authors to follow standard recommendations for the publications of a given type of study. Following the guidelines in Table 2.7 is not only a prerequisite for getting a study accepted but also useful advice to help authors in writing.

Among the items in the guideline for drafting manuscripts, one of the vital things is to critically evaluate the study and interpret the results accordingly. A useful preliminary task is to carefully read the title and abstract of the report to decide if the trials' findings are relevant and hence to determine whether the report is trustworthy. Furthermore, the real test trial's validity lies in careful look through the methods section. The design of a trial largely determines whether an unbiased and objective therapeutic comparison can be made. In the discussion of the report, the strengths and weaknesses of the study as compared to other studies should be addressed.

Table 2.7 List of reporting guidelines

Name of the statement	Applicable study type	Website/resources
CONSORT	Randomized controlled trials	www.consort-statement.org
STRICTA	Randomized controlled trials for acupuncture	www.stricta.info
STROBE	Observational studies	www.strobe-statement.org
STARD	Diagnostic accuracy studies	www.stard-statement.org
TREND	Nonrandomized studies for behavioral and public health interventions	www.cdc.gov/trendstatement
SPIRIT	Trial protocol	www.spirit-statement.org
COREQ	Qualitative studies	www.equator-network.org
PRISMA	Systematic reviews and metaanalysis	www.prisma-statement.org
MOOSE	Systematic review of observational studies	JAMA 2008, 283 (15) [18]

2.2.4.3 Publishing the Manuscript

After submitting the manuscript to a journal, the authors should wait for the first decision made by editors on whether the manuscript merits external peer review. The first decision may take days or weeks. Hopefully, the manuscript would be sent to two or more external peer reviewers and the peer review process may take months. There are three possibilities to the submission, be accepted, be requested to have revision, or be rejected. If the decision letter requests a revised version of the manuscript, one should forward the decision letter to all coauthors. Besides amending the manuscript, a response letter is needed for resubmission. It is acceptable not to follow all recommendations if you explain why. Each question/ point raised by peer reviewers in the response letter should be answered/ addressed in a cooperative and unambiguous manner. Even if the submission were rejected by the journal, authors should try to consider rationally the problems and the chances of getting the manuscript accepted elsewhere.

Acknowledgments Huijuan Cao was supported by the 2015 Beijing Organization Department Outstanding Talented Person Project (Grant No. 2015000020124G083); Both Huijuan Cao and Jianping Liu were supported by a Construction Project from the Beijing Municipal Education Commission.

References

1. Liu JP, et al. Study methods of evidence-based Chinese medicine. Beijing: People's Health Press; 2010. pp. 21–4.
2. Witt CM, Linde K. Clinical research in complementary and integrative medicine: a practical training book. Hackerbrucke: Urban and Fischer; 2012. pp. 65–74.
3. Pocock SJ. Clinical trials: a practical approach. John Wiley and Sons; 1983. pp. 97–9.
4. Cao H, et al. Medicinal cupping therapy in 30 patients with fibromyalgia: a case series observation. Forsch Komplementmed. 2011;18:112–6.
5. Zhang L, et al. Prevalence of chronic kidney disease in China: a cross-sectional survey. Lancet. 2012;379:815–22.
6. Hsu PC, et al. Integrating traditional Chinese medicine healthcare into diabetes care by reducing the risk of developing kidney failure among type 2 diabetic patients: a population-based case control study. J Ethnopharmacol. 2014;156:358–64.
7. Su SY, et al. Use of Chinese medicine correlates negatively with the consumption of conventional medicine and medical cost in patients with uterine fibroids: a population-based retrospective cohort study in Taiwan. BMC Complement Altern Med. 2015;15(1):129.
8. Zhang CS, et al. Ear acupressure for perennial allergic rhinitis: a multicenter randomized controlled trial. Am J Rhinol Allergy. 2014;28(4):e152–7.
9. Witt CM, et al. Homoeopathic versus conventional therapy for atopic eczema in children: medical and economic results. Dermatology. 2009;219(4):329–40.
10. Liu JP, Chen KJ. The guideline development team. Methodology guideline for clinical study investigating traditional Chinese medicine and integrative medicine. Complement Ther Med. 2015;23:751–6.
11. Kim SY. Comparative effectiveness research in primary practice. Korean J Fam Med. 2012;33:329.

12. Mayer D. Essential evidence-based medicine (second edition). Cambridge: Cambridge University Press; 2010. pp. 367–78.
13. Higgins JPT, Green S (editors). Cochrane handbook for systematic reviews of interventions version 5.1.0 [updated March 2011]. The Cochrane Collaboration, 2011. Available from www.cochrane-handbook.org.
14. Cao H, et al. Cupping therapy for acute and chronic pain management: a systematic review of randomized clinical trials. J Tradit Chin Med Sci 2014; 1:49e61.
15. Manheimer E, Wieland S, Kimbrough E, Cheng K, Berman BM. Evidence from the cochrane collaboration for traditional Chinese medicine therapies. J Altern Complement Med. 2009;15 (9):1001–14.
16. Cao H, et al. Using a partially randomized patient preference study design to evaluate the therapeutic effect of acupuncture and cupping therapy for fibromyalgia: study protocol for a partially randomized controlled trial. Trials. 2014;15:280.
17. Liu JP, et al. Prospective registration, bias risk and outcome-reporting bias in randomised clinical trials of traditional Chinese medicine: an empirical methodological study. BMJ Open. 2013; 3(7):pii:e002968.
18. Stroup DF, et al. Meta-analysis of observational studies in epidemiology: a proposal for reporting. JAMA. 2000;283(15):2008–12.

Chapter 3
Effectiveness Assessment of Chinese Medicine in Clinical Research

Liming Lu, Xinfeng Guo and Zehuai Wen

Abstract The purpose of effectiveness assessment is to assist health care providers and patients to make informed decisions that will improve health care. How to assess the effectiveness of Chinese medicine (CM) scientifically is a critical issue and needs to be resolved. We summarize the advances in outcome research into the effectiveness assessment of CM in this chapter. For principles of effectiveness assessment, we need to select outcome measures according to the research purpose and synthetically consider evidence of randomized controlled trials and well-designed observational studies. The outcome categories include primary outcome, secondary outcome, composite outcome, surrogate outcome, and patient-reported outcomes (PROs). The advantages, disadvantages, and function comparison of primary and secondary outcomes should be identified. Composite outcomes are often applied to clinical trials in case of unavailable or impractical primary outcomes. The composite outcomes can also capture the multidimensional nature of disease, seek a comprehensive response to intervention, and thus could be especially important for complex intervention including CM. The development and validation of a composite outcome should be through rigorous scientific research design and statistical model. When the secondary outcome is confirmed to be associated with the true clinical outcome and completely reflect the net effect of treatment on the outcome, this secondary outcome can also be the surrogate outcome. Although the definition of the surrogate outcome has been proposed, the application is limited currently. PROs are supposed to highlight the features and superiority of CM in clinical effectiveness assessment. Developing a new PRO instrument based on CM treatment nature by the standard procedures is feasible to be commonly recognized and accepted in biomedicine. Based on the integration of

L. Lu · X. Guo · Z. Wen (✉)
Key Unit of Methodology in Clinical Research, Guangdong Provincial Hospital of Chinese Medicine, Guangzhou University of Chinese Medicine, Guangzhou 510120, China
e-mail: wenzh@gzucm.edu.cn

L. Lu
e-mail: lulimingleon@126.com

X. Guo
e-mail: drguoxinfeng@163.com

S. Leung and H. Hu (eds.), *Evidence-based Research Methods for Chinese Medicine*, DOI 10.1007/978-981-10-2290-6_3

domestic and foreign research view in recent years, we systematically describe both retrospective and prospective effectiveness assessment studies. Finally, we illustrate the outcome selection by examples. In summary, we must clearly recognize the differences in primary, secondary, and surrogate outcomes, and choose the appropriate outcome measures according to the study purposes, study models, and CM characteristics.

Keywords Effectiveness assessment · Outcome research · Chinese medicine

3.1 Introduction

Chinese medicine (CM) has been used in China and other eastern Asia countries for many years, and has been widely popular among patients in many other countries [1]. Faith and popularity of CM are mainly depended on its efficacy. However, this does not mean that all of CM therapies are effective. CM therapies still need to be rigorously evaluated exactly as any other interventions. According to Tang JL, "research in CM should adopt a recognized and efficacy driven approach to show efficacy in humans" [2]. But how to show or evaluate the effectiveness of CM interventions? In our viewpoint, this issue does not have principal difference compared with other interventions of biomedicine; all we have to do is considering the characteristics of CM with the exception of outcomes assessment.

This chapter presents a summary of outcome research in the effectiveness assessment of CM aiming to benefit the researcher performing a rigorous and scientific effectiveness assessment study. In particular, this chapter is designed to help researchers to (a) identify the factors influencing clinical effectiveness; (b) master the relationship between effectiveness assessment and outcome measurement and principles of effectiveness assessment for CM interventions; (c) recognize the discrimination during primary, secondary, surrogate, and patient-reported outcomes (PROs) to choose the appropriate outcome measurements according to the study purpose, study model, and CM characteristics; and (d) understand the types of study design and their data analysis methods in effectiveness assessment research of CM.

3.2 Definition of Clinical Effectiveness of Interventions

Clinical effectiveness is a measure of the extent to which a clinical intervention, when deployed in the field in routine circumstances, does what it is intended to do for a specific population [1]. The purpose of effectiveness assessment is to assist health care providers and patients to decide how to improve health care [2–4]. It is believed that clinical effectiveness is the basis of the existence and development of CM. Thus, how to assess the effectiveness of CM scientifically is a critical issue to be resolved.

3.3 Factors Influencing Clinical Effectiveness: Risk of Bias and PICOS in Clinical Trials

Effectiveness inferences from RCTs can be weaken by flaws in design, conduct, analyses, and reporting, affecting the credibility of the true intervention effect [5]. Therefore, we should know the PICOS (Participants, Intervention, Comparison, Outcome, and Study design) model of clinical research and factors affecting clinical effectiveness.

On the one hand, we need to identify the risk of bias in clinical researches including several biases: selection bias, performance bias, detection bias, attrition bias, reporting bias, and other bias [6]. A clear understanding of risk of bias can benefit the quality control of the whole process during the trial and inducing confident results. In addition, systematic reviews can obtain reliable conclusions after considering the potential flaws of the included studies. Specially, for the randomized controlled trials (RCTs) of CM, it is strongly recommended to use appropriate allocation method. Randomization is used frequently at the level of individual patients and dynamic allocation procedures may be used as an alternative [4]. The final choice depends on the study design [7]. Blinded outcome assessment is applied to reduce bias when outcome judgement may be affected by subjective bodies. Recommendations for blinding the treatment can be found in the guidelines developed in the European Union funded GP-TCM project [8]. Sample size should be calculated in the trials' design phase, on the basis of the main outcome and the minimum clinically important difference (MCID) from previous published reports. For subgroup analysis, it is interesting when different CM diagnosis patterns and patients who are naïve/non-naïve to CM are considered. Although it is still difficult to incorporate the concept of *zheng* (syndrome) differentiation into the RCTs currently due to methodological limitations, further analyses can be carried out for different *zheng* differentiations if sample size permits.

On the other hand, we should establish the criteria or definitions for every part of the PICOS setting. For patient included criteria, both Western medicine and CM approaches should be applied to clearly define the study disease and patients' conditions. A clear, comprehensive, and well-recognized CM diagnosis patterns would benefit the exploratory analysis and hypothesis generation for future studies. Some measures should be taken to strengthen the reliability of *zheng* differentiations of CM (assessing inter-rater agreement and providing training). A big enough sample size is required to ensure the internal homogeneity. For the selection of intervention, evidence-based practice of CM is addressed by available reports, protocols, clinical data, or formal consensus procedures. Pharmaceutical composition and dosage are fixed for herbal decoction to ensure reproducibility. We should take some measures to ensure the quality and stability of herbal drugs. For example, the herbal decoction can be dried at low-temperature into granules after the compound is decocted and concentrated. For non-pharmaceutical interventions, such as acupuncture, moxibustion, massage, and tai-chi, quality control is necessarily conducted in many processes (therapist experience, points' selection, and operation methods). For comparison, evidence, guidelines, or broad expert consensus are also addressed during the selection process. Placebo is appropriate for the control group when there still lacks effective treatment and it will not harm the patients without medication in short term. Decoction placebo can be made of pigments, bitter elements, and special flavor to imitate the test drug's color and odor. A pretest should be performed to guarantee this placebo is inactive in treatment and works on blinding. Acupuncture placebo includes acupuncture in sham points, sham needles in true points, and special double-blinded devices. Gentle touch can be used as control for massage and gymnastics. Similar exercises can be used as control tai-chi.

3.4 Considering CM Characteristics

3.4.1 Effectiveness Assessment and Outcome Measurement

Clinical epidemiology engages in outcome research [9, 10]. Generally, the purposes, methods, and principles of clinical assessment are consistent with those of outcome research and incorporated into the scope of outcome research [9]. It is believed that appropriate outcome measures are important to clinical research of CM. First, patient-centered main outcome measures comply with CM therapy's characteristics. CM is generally considered as holistic medicine; thus, it has advantages of adjusting the whole body's functions and self-feeling, but the CM's effectiveness is generally moderate and slower than that of allopathic way of modern Western medicine. How to select the appropriate outcome measures complying with therapy's characteristics of CM is still a research hotspot. Second, opposite conclusions can be drawn using different outcome endpoints [11, 12]. CM's effectiveness should be confirmed by commonly recognized measures [13]. Many institutions, such as NIH and Cochrane Collaboration, are demanding the clinical effectiveness from the appropriate outcomes.

In order to know the status of outcome research in CM, our research team has investigated the outcomes used in the RCTs of CM in several conditions. Taking chronic obstructive pulmonary disease (COPD) for example [14]. We showed that of the 12 outcomes, pulmonary function [forced expiratory volume in 1 second (FEV1)], St. George's Respiratory Questionnaire (SGRQ), modified Medical Research Council (mMRC), 6-minute walk distance (6MWDS), exacerbation frequency, and adverse events were assessed as the critical outcomes, the composite outcomes such as the response rate, a combination of the improvement of symptoms, signs, and laboratory indexes were rated as low importance for decision making because of problems in methodology. The rest of outcomes were important but not critical. Of the 539 included articles, 213 (40 %) used lung function to evaluate the treatment effect and 19 (4 %) used SGRQ, while 426 articles (including 21 different judgement standards) used the response rate (total effectiveness rate, TER), accounting for 79 % of all clinical trials for COPD. These results informed us that only a small number of RCTs of CM for COPD used appropriate outcomes. In another case of CM treatment for chronic urticarial, in which no suitable primary clinical endpoint was available, almost all trials used the response rate (TER), which were not explicit and validated and rated as of limited importance for clinical decision making.

3.4.2 Principles of Effectiveness Assessment for CM Interventions

Outcome assessment focuses on selecting appropriate outcome into scientific measurement practice of CM's effectiveness. Only the primary outcomes with direct effects on patients can measure the true effectiveness of CM [12]. Based on the characteristics of CM theory and clinical practice, Lai SL proposed a comprehensive "CM effectiveness assessment framework" [15], suggesting (1) commonly accepted effectiveness measures; (2) measurements of CM syndrome-/pattern-related symptoms or PROs; and (3) quality of life with universal- and disease-specific evaluation items embodying the characteristics of CM. Afterwards, researchers continued the development of clinical effectiveness assessment system with CM characteristics [15–18]. In summary, effectiveness assessment of CM contains (1) biology outcomes and their changes reflecting the effects of CM; (2) patient-reported outcomes (PROs), proxy-reported outcomes, and physician-reported outcomes (outcome assessment by patients, their families, caregivers, or health care workers); (3) safety assessment: adverse event reports and the causality evaluation related to CM; and (4) health economics, e.g., efficiency measurement and evaluation of CM.

In addition, depending on the research purposes, the effectiveness assessment of CM may use different outcome measures to assess a variety of diseases and CM syndromes. For example, researchers and policymakers often distinguish between the efficacy and the effectiveness of an intervention. Efficacy trials (explanatory trials) determine whether an intervention produces the expected result under ideal circumstances. However, effectiveness trials (pragmatic trials) measure the effects under "real world" clinical settings [19, 20]. Thus, outcome selection should meet the different characteristics and purposes of efficacy or effectiveness trials.

Sometimes, it takes time to demonstrate the therapeutic effect of an intervention. Specially, in terms of CM, the research process may include case accumulation, observational studies, exploratory research, confirmatory trials, and reevaluation studies. From the perspective of evidence-based medicine (EBM), this is also a research process of various types of associated evidence to demonstrate the efficacy or effectiveness. RCT is not the only effectiveness assessment of CM. Well-designed observational studies can provide some useful implications. Effectiveness assessment of CM should synthesise the evidence from both RCTs and observational studies.

3.4.3 Primary and Secondary Outcomes

In clinical trials, primary and secondary outcomes are measured over the course of the disease, and treatment benefits can be evaluated on all of them. The primary outcome is a clinical endpoint that fully characterizes clinically the effect of treatment and assists the researchers to make a claim for the treatment [21]. Besides, the primary outcome is used to perform the sample size calculation to detect a specified clinical benefit. Sometimes, limited time and resources may force the investigators to use alternative outcomes, such as secondary outcome [22]. For examples, it is not possible to observe the duration of survival as the ultimate outcome in chronic diseases due to the prolonged period of follow-up. Compared to the primary outcome, the secondary outcome is not sufficient to characterize fully the benefit or to support a claim for a treatment effect but provides additional clinical characterization of the treatment effect [21]. Table 3.1 describes the comparison of primary and secondary outcomes.

The outcome selection is dependent upon the research purpose to provide a reference for decision making of clinical treatment. Thus, it is suitable to endorse more direct and relevant outcomes to measure the treatment effect, such as endpoints of survival, mortality, diminished capacity, and disability level. For example, in the effectiveness assessment of artemisinin for falciparum malaria, mortality rate is the most suitable primary outcome related to the treatment effect. By contrast, for the exploratory research focusing on the pathogenesis mechanism of falciparum malaria, the endpoints reflecting artemisinin's interference of falciparum malaria's life history (not mortality rate) should be more related to the pathogenesis mechanism.

Besides, the purpose and/or hypothesis of an RCT of CM determines the study model, which can be categorized as the Western medicine disease-oriented model, the CM *zheng*-oriented model, or the integrated model [23]. The outcome selection should be consistent with both the research purpose and the study model. For the Western medicine disease-oriented model, the outcomes should be disease-oriented as the study aims to determine whether CM can relief the targeted disease. In this situation, Western medicine's symptoms, signs, and examinations may be the primary and/or secondary outcome measures. Similarly, for the CM model, CM-specific *zheng*-oriented endpoints are the covariates to determine whether CM can benefit the *zheng*. For the integrated model, both CM-oriented and Western medicine-oriented endpoints could be the primary and/or secondary outcomes [24].

For the selection among similar outcomes, we should comprehensively consider and discriminate the outcomes' objectivity, stability, sensitivity, and specificity in

Table 3.1 Comparison of primary outcome and secondary outcome [12]

	Properties	Advantages	Disadvantages	Functions
Primary outcome	True outcome for the disease or interventional effect	Characterize the true effect of treatment with less bias	Appear late; need more time and large sample size; easily be interfered by bias	Verify the effect of treatment and promote its application
Secondary/surrogate outcome	Not true clinical outcome, not sufficient to characterize fully the benefit or risk of treatment	Appear in early; reduce time and sample size; more objective; less variation; easy to measure	Easily be interfered by bias without strict evaluation of validity	Explore the treatment mechanism; test the treatment effect in some conditions

the specific disease and the CM *zheng*. In fact, different roles show different preferences in outcome measures. For example, patients concern whether their body function or self-feeling can be improved; thus, the endpoints reflecting diminished capacity, self-feeling, or quality of life (QOL) are more suitable for the measurement. Practitioners concern whether the patients' pathological damages can be reversed; thus, the endpoints of their physiology and biochemistry are preferred for the measurement. And health authorities pay more attention to health economic evaluations.

Currently, many clinical trials aim to determine the effectiveness of interventions mainly depending on the improvement of specific disease-related biomarkers and medical examinations. These biomarkers play important roles in the treatment effects and mechanisms, but they are secondary outcomes. Only the primary outcomes can provide sufficient evidence to characterize clinically treatment effects. Especially, only the sensitive outcomes characterized with *zheng* differentiation of CM are indispensable for scientific and systematic assessment of CM's effectiveness.

3.4.4 Composite Outcome

Most CM treatments are complex interventions, and thus the mechanism of therapeutic effects of CM are obviously different from that of powerful single-targeted allopathic Western medicine. Therefore, the composite outcomes which can reflect the multidimensional overall changes of conditions are scientifically significant to comprehensive evaluation of clinical effectiveness of CM. Composite outcomes are often applied to clinical trials for many reasons: unavailable or impractical primary outcomes, or to capture the multidimensional nature of diseases and responses of interventions. Composite outcomes can usually reduce sample size by increasing outcome rates, but also cause concerns of multiplicity for testing many outcomes, and other competing risks including uninterpretability when heterogeneity exists in a composite outcome [25].

For example, FEV1 is often used to evaluate the severity of chronic obstructive pulmonary disease (COPD). However, patients with COPD have systemic manifestations that are not reflected by the FEV1. Celli et al. developed a composite outcome which can better assess the respiratory and systemic expressions of COPD [26]. They first evaluated 207 patients and selected four factors from 12 factors which had strongest correlations with the 1-year mortality in the cohort: the body mass index (B), the degree of airflow obstruction (O), dyspnea (D), and exercise capacity (E). With these factors, they constructed the BODE index with a multidimensional 10-point scale (the higher the scores, the worse the health). They prospectively validated the index in a cohort of 625 patients, with death from any cause and from respiratory causes as the primary outcome (golden standard variable). Empirical model, Cox proportional hazards regression analyses, and the C statistic were used to build and test the BODE index. The research found that the BODE index as a composite outcome is better than the FEV1 or any other index alone in predicting the risk of death among COPD patients.

Development and validation of a composite outcome should be through rigorous research design and statistical model. The researcher should evaluate the sensitivity and specificity of the composite outcome correlated with the primary outcome in a prospective study. For the development of composite outcome for the complex intervention, the main components of complex intervention and the function of each component should be understood thoroughly.

3.4.5 Surrogate Outcome and Patient-Reported Outcome

When the secondary outcome is confirmed to be related to the true clinical outcome and fully capture the net effect of treatment on the clinical outcome (in a prospective study), this secondary outcome can be called a successful surrogate outcome [27]. A surrogate outcome of clinical trial is a laboratory measurement or a physical sign used as a substitute for a clinically meaningful endpoint that measures directly how a patient feels, functions, or survives. Changes induced by a therapy on a surrogate outcome are expected to reflect changes in a clinically meaningful endpoint [28]. Surrogate outcomes are applied when the endpoint of interest is too difficult and/or expensive to measure routinely, as a substitute which is sufficiently correlated with the true clinical outcome [29]. Table 3.1 describes the comparison of primary and surrogate outcomes.

Figure 3.1 describes the setting of surrogate outcomes' application. Specifically, the surrogate outcome is in the only causal pathway of the disease process mediating the intervention's entire effect on the true clinical outcome [28]. Previous examples of surrogate outcomes are tumor regression in trials of cancer therapy, suppression of ventricular arrhythmias or reduction in cholesterol level or blood pressure in cardiology trials, increased CD4 cell counts, or decreased viral load measures for trials of human immunodeficiency virus (HIV) infection or AIDS. However, cardiac output, cholesterol levels, ventricular arrhythmias, and tumor shrinkage were sometimes not successful when used as the surrogate outcome in cardiologic disorder or cancer measurements. Some considerations must be taken into the clinical trial when the surrogate outcome is applied. First, the surrogate outcome may not be the real predictor of clinical outcome. It can measure the mechanism of the intervention for the disease but cannot provide all the information related to the treatment and subsequent impact. For example, the surrogate outcome is positive but the clinical outcome is negative. Second, it is not feasible to compare the surrogate outcome and the side effect, leading to the difficulty of weighting the effectiveness of intervention. Although the definition of the surrogate outcome has been proposed, the application is limited currently.

The efficacy and safety of CM has been practiced through experience rather than scientific measurements. Patient-reported outcomes (PROs) are supposed to show the features and superiority of CM in clinical effectiveness assessment. PROs refer to patients' self-reported outcomes in the context of health care, including their living environment, health conditions, and treatment [30]. PROs include not only health status and quality of life but also reports on satisfaction with treatment and care, adherence to prescribed regimens, and any other outcome evaluation obtained directly from patients through interviews, self-completed questionnaires, diaries, or other data collection tools such as handheld devices and web-based forms [30–33]. In other words, PROs include, but not limited to, health-related quality of life, symptoms, patient satisfaction with treatment, functional status, psychological well-being, and treatment adherence [34]. In fact, many subjective symptoms, such as diet, sleep, and pain, collected by questioning, are the foundation for medical diagnosis and treatment of CM. The efficacy of CM in treating the disease is to intervene the pathological mechanisms of all signs and symptoms. By contrast, the

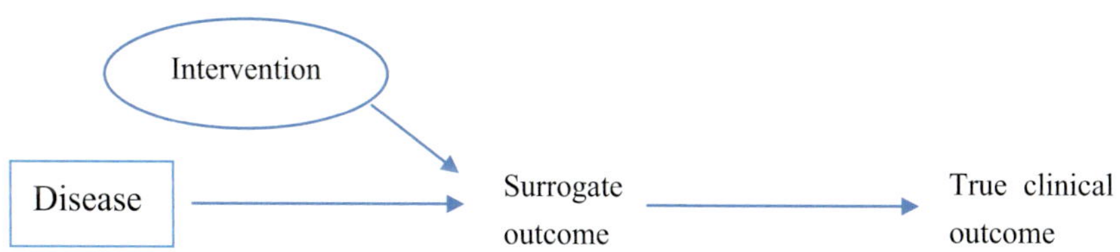

Fig. 3.1 Pathway of valid surrogate outcome mediating intervention with true clinical outcome [28]

inefficacy means no improvement of symptoms and signs. Thus, PROs is important to CM diagnosis and treatment [35].

However, it is not suitable to use some currently available PROs instruments in evaluating treatment of CM or integrative medicine. For example, the present health-related quality of life (HRQOL) instruments based on Western medical knowledge cannot meet the requirement of expressing special characteristics of CM treatment efficacy. It has been feasible to develop a new HRQOL instrument based on CM and Chinese culture by the standard and scientific procedures. The psychometric properties of the instrument are satisfactory to detect important changes in clinical studies. It is useful in both Chinese and integrative medicine [36].

3.5 Types of Design and Methods of Data Analysis

Based on the integration of domestic and foreign research in recent years, we systematically classify the types of study design and their data analysis in CM as follows: effectiveness assessment study of retrospective data (clinical medical records; previous clinical research data) and prospective effectiveness assessment study (disease registers; longitudinal study; RCTs).

3.5.1 Retrospective Effectiveness Assessment Studies

3.5.1.1 Clinical Medical Records

Structured electronic medical record sharing system needs to be constructed first. Clinical diagnosis and treatment information can be converted into structured data from medical records. We can connect the data resources of patient-centered hospital information system (HIS), biochemical test systems, and imaging system. Clinical information of diseases and *zheng* in CM can be comprehensively collected by studies of longitudinal observational studies. For statistical analysis, some issues should be considered include different *zheng* of the same disease, different diseases of the same *zheng*, and different diseases associated with *zheng* can be compared. By combing technologies of mathematics and informatics, including data mining, quantitative synthesis, and modeling the biological information of *zheng* in CM can be better understood.

3.5.1.2 Previous Clinical Research

Databases provide helpful information on existing CM trials (for example, Oregon College of Oriental Medicine for Acupuncture (AcuTrials®) [37], New England School of Acupuncture (NESA) Database [38], Chinese BioMedical Literature

Database (CBM) [39], China Network Knowledge Infrastructure (CNKI) [40], and Chinese Scientific Journals Database (VIP) [41]). Besides, it is necessary to form CM databases of clinical research based on previous clinical trials and develop the guidance to encourage CM clinical investigators to share their raw data. Meta-analysis can be applied to perform direct and indirect comparisons of different effects of CM and screen the optimal treatment. Decision trees, association rules, support vector machines, and artificial neural networks can be used to analyze the past data to identify the associated factors of CM or Western medicine, investigate the possible roles of CM, and improve existing knowledge.

3.5.2 *Prospective Effectiveness Assessment Studies*

Deficiencies of historical data mentioned above is may be that limited variables the researcher is interested in and some necessary analysis hard to perform. Thus, it is necessary to perform the prospective effectiveness assessment study to satisfy the following requirements:

3.5.2.1 Disease Registers and Longitudinal Studies

Good literature reviews and preliminary discussions can be performed before designing the questionnaire. We should fully consider the patients' related impact factors, including general demographics, lifestyle, medical history, physical examination, laboratory and imaging studies, past therapies (included CM), and contextual factors. A CM structured questionnaire serves as the carrier of clinical information data, which should be based on standardized terminology of clinical data interchange standards consortium (CDISC). For statistical analysis, the propensity score method can be used to balance the comparability among characteristic variables of different groups with given and known covariates [42, 43]. When there are a number of potential confounders unknown in the real world, the instrumental variable method can be balanced against the known and unknown variables. This method can handle the relationship between covariates and the result of factors and explore a variable that is related to the explanatory variables but has nothing to do with the results. Its purpose is to give an unbiased estimate of the effect. However, it would be difficult to find the right instrumental variable.

3.5.2.2 RCTs

Research should clearly describe the diagnostic criteria in terms of Western medicine and CM; settings should be based on valid evidence; implementation details of acupuncture, qigong, or tai-chi should be declared; herbal formulation, dosage, and cost should be considered; appropriate random allocation method should be applied; and the implementation of blinding, sample size calculation and preferences, and expectations of the subjects should be evaluated. In order to assess the effectiveness of treatments, we should compare the benefits and harms of the treatment [44].

3.6 Case Study

We give one of our studies to illustrate the decision process of outcome selection. This study was designed to address the effectiveness of combined Chinese medicine (CM-)-based psychotherapy and Chinese herbal medicine (CHM) in the treatment of menopausal syndrome [45]. Many females of menopausal syndrome suffer from a considerable variety of symptoms, including hot flashes, night sweats, menstrual irregularities, vaginal dryness, depression, nervous tension, palpitations, and others. Conventional hormone replacement therapy (HRT) cannot relieve all of the symptoms. CM-based psychotherapy refers to any form of therapeutic interaction or treatment that aims to increase the individual's sense of well-being. Favorable outcomes should be associated with psychological symptoms, such as menopausal syndrome.

As mentioned above, the efficacy of CM for the disease is to eliminate all signs and symptoms. Thus, the PROs is important to CM diagnosis and treatment evaluation. For the CM model, a CM-specific *zheng*-oriented endpoint is more appropriate to be the primary outcome. Thus, we chose the Kupperman Index (KI) and the menopause-specific quality of life (MENQOL) as the primary outcomes to directly measure the treatment effect. We believed these measurements could clinically characterize the treatment effect and support a regulatory claim for the treatment. The secondary outcomes included serum levels of FSH and E_2 and symptom relief. These biological and pathological endpoints play important roles in determining the interventions' effects and possible mechanism.

3.7 Summary

How to assess the effectiveness of CM in scientific manner is still a critical issue in practice. We focused on the consideration of how to choose the appropriate outcomes to clinically characterize the effects of CM treatment and possible mechanism. In recent years, more and more clinical trials of CM are emerging with concerns of study quality [46]. It seems that some issues should be resolved by better research. First, in terms of CM, the research may be case accumulation, observational studies, exploratory research, confirmatory trials, and reevaluation studies. RCT is not the only preference for effectiveness assessment of CM. Well-designed observational studies can sometimes provide useful implications. Effectiveness assessment of CM should synthesize the evidence from both RCTs and observational studies. Second, we must clearly recognize the differences in primary, secondary, and surrogate outcomes, and choose the appropriate outcome measures according to the study purposes, study models, and CM characteristics.

References

1. Last JM. A dictionary of epidemiology. New York: Oxford University Press; 2001.
2. Takeshita J, Gelfand JM. Comparative effectiveness research: what it is and how to assess its quality. Wiley; 2014. pp. 66–70.
3. Witt CM, Aickin M, Baca T, Cherkin D, Haan MN, Hammerschlag R, Hao JJ, Kaplan GA, Lao L, McKay T, Pierce B, Riley D, Ritenbaugh C, Thorpe K, Tunis S, Weissberg J. Berman BM. Effectiveness Guidance Documents Collaborators. Effectiveness guidance document (EGD) for acupuncture research—a consensus document for conducting trials. BMC Complement Altern Med. 2012;12:148.
4. Witt CM, Aickin M, Cherkin D, Che CT, Elder C, Flower A, Hammerschlag R, Liu JP, Lao L, Phurrough S, Ritenbaugh C, Rubin LH, Schnyer R, Wayne PM, Withers SR, Zhao-Xiang B, Young J. Berman BM. Collaborators. Effectiveness Guidance Document (EGD) for Chinese medicine trials: a consensus document. Trials. 2014;15:169.
5. Wood L, Egger M, Gluud LL, Schulz KF, Jüni P, Altman DG, Gluud C, Martin RM, Wood AJ, Sterne JA. Empirical evidence of bias in treatment effect estimates in controlled trials with different interventions and outcomes: meta-epidemiological study. BMJ. 2008;336:601–5.
6. Higgins JP, Altman DG, Gøtzsche PC, Jüni P, Moher D, Oxman AD, Savovic J, Schulz KF, Weeks L. Sterne JA; Cochrane Bias Methods Group; Cochrane Statistical Methods Group. The Cochrane Collaboration's tool for assessing risk of bias in randomised trials. BMJ. 2011;343:d5928.
7. Taves DR. Rank-minimization with a two-step analysis should replace randomization in clinical trials. J Clin Epidemiol. 2012;65:3–6.
8. Good Practice in Traditional Chinese Medicine Research Association. GP-TCM project; 2015. http://www.gp-tcm.org/zh.
9. Wen Z. Effectiveness assessment and its research policy of Chinese medicine. Chin J Integr Tradit W Med. 2011;4:452–4.
10. Weiss NS. Clinical epidemiology—disease outcomes research. Beijing: Beijing University Press; 2014.
11. De Gruttola VG, Clax P, DeMets DL, Downing GJ, Ellenberg SS, Friedman L, Gail MH, Prentice R, Wittes J, Zeger SL. Considerations in the evaluation of surrogate endpoints in clinical trials. Summary of a National Institutes of Health workshop. Control Clin Trials. 2001;22:485–502.
12. Guo X. Selection and application of outcome indicators in effectiveness assessment of Chinese medicine. J Guangzhou Univ Tradit Chin Med. 2002;4:251–5.
13. Levin JS, Glass TA, Kushi LH, Schuck JR, Steele L, Jonas WB. Quantitative methods in research on complementary and alternative medicine. A methodological manifesto. NIH Office of Alternative Medicine. Med Care. 1997;35:1079–94.
14. Guo X, Liu S, Yang L, Wu L. The importance of GRADE for TCM clinical research on COPD: from the perspective of outcomes. Methodology conference of evidence-based clinical practice guideline and clinical pathway in traditional Chinese medicine (TCM) and GRADE in systematic reviews and guideline development workshops (Guangzhou). 2015;77–82.
15. Lai S, Hu J, Guo X. Evidence-based medicine and clinical study of traditional Chinese medicine. J Guangzhou Univ Tradit Chin Med. 2000;17:1–8.

16. Liang X. Problems and thinking about the effectiveness assessment of traditional Chinese medicine. China J Tradit Chin Med Pharm. 2006;21:37–9.
17. Chen S, Liang W. Discussion on the application of index of TCM syndromes in effectiveness assessment of traditional Chinese medicine. J New Chin Med. 2008;40:113–5.
18. Liu Q, Liu C, Yuan H. Establishing the system of effectiveness assessment in line with self-developed demands of TCM. Lishizhen Med Mater Med Res. 2010;21:1279–80.
19. Godwin M, Ruhland L, Casson I, MacDonald S, Delva D, Birtwhistle R, Lam M, Seguin R. Pragmatic controlled clinical trials in primary care: the struggle between external and internal validity. BMC Med Res Methodol. 2003;3:28.
20. Witt CM, Manheimer E, Hammerschlag R, Lüdtke R, Lao L, Tunis SR, Berman BM. How well do randomized trials inform decision making: systematic review using comparative effectiveness research measures on acupuncture for back pain. PLoS ONE. 2012;7:e32399.
21. O'Neill RT. Secondary endpoints cannot be validly analyzed if the primary endpoint does not demonstrate clear statistical significance. Control Clin Trials. 1997;18:550–6, 561–7.
22. Buyse M, Molenberghs G. Criteria for the validation of surrogate endpoints in randomized experiments. Biometrics. 1998;54:1014–29.
23. Zheng S, Bian Z, Li Y. How to explain the methodological rationale of randomized controlled trials of traditional Chinese medicine? Zhongguo Xun Zheng Yi Xue Za Zhi. 2008;8:152–4.
24. Bian ZX, Moher D, Li YP, Wu TX, Dagenais S, Cheng CW, Li J, Li TQ. Appropriately selecting and concisely reporting the outcome measures of randomized controlled trials of traditional Chinese medicine. Zhong Xi Yi Jie He Xue Bao. 2008;6:771–5.
25. Pogue J, Thabane L, Devereaux PJ, Yusuf S. Testing for heterogeneity among the components of a binary composite outcome in a clinical trial. BMC Med Res Methodol. 2010;10:49.
26. Celli BR, Cote CG, Marin JM, Casanova C, Montes de Oca M, Mendez RA, Pinto Plata V, Cabral HJ. The body-mass index, airflow obstruction, dyspnea, and exercise capacity index in chronic obstructive pulmonary disease. N Engl J Med. 2004;350:1005–12.
27. Prentice RL. Surrogate endpoints in clinical trials: definition and operational criteria. Stat Med. 1989;8:431–40.
28. Fleming TR, Demets DL. Surrogate end points in clinical trials: are we being misled? Ann Intern Med. 1996;125:605–13.
29. Ellenberg S, Hamilton JM. Surrogate endpoints in clinical trials: cancer. Stat Med. 1989;8:405–13.
30. Zhao L, Chan K. Patient-reported outcomes (PROs): an approach to evaluate treatment efficacy of Chinese medicine or integrative medicine. Chin J Integr Med. 2005;11:151–3.
31. Kyte DG, Draper H, Ives J, Liles C, Gheorghe A, Calvert M. Patient reported outcomes (PROs) in clinical trials: is 'in-trial' guidance lacking? A systematic review. PLoS ONE. 2013;8:e60684.
32. Weldring T, Smith SM. Patient-reported outcomes (PROs) and patient-reported outcome measures (PROMs). Health Serv Insights. 2013;6:61–8.
33. Snyder CF, Jensen RE, Segal JB, Wu AW. Patient-reported outcomes (PROs): putting the patient perspective in patient-centered outcomes research. Med Care. 2013;51:S73–9.
34. Acquadro C, Berzon R, Dubois D, Leidy NK, Marquis P, Revicki D, Rothman M. PRO Harmonization Group. Incorporating the patient's perspective into drug development and communication: an ad hoc task force report of the patient-reported outcomes (PRO) Harmonization group meeting at the food and drug administration, February 16, 2001. Value Health. 2003;6:522–31.
35. Wang J, He QY. Thinking on how to construct the system of Chinese medicine efficacy evaluation for coronary heart disease angina pectoris. Chin J Integr Med. 2010;16:75–8.
36. Zhao L, Chan K. Building a bridge for integrating Chinese medicine into conventional healthcare: observations drawn from the development of the Chinese quality of life instrument. Am J Chin Med. 2005;33:897–902.
37. Oregon College of Oriental Medicine. AcuTrials Database; 2016. http://library.ocom.edu/.
38. New England School of Acupuncture. NESA Database; 2016. http://www.nesa.edu/research.

39. Chinese Academy of Medical Sciences. Chinese BioMedical Literature Database. 2016; http://sinomed.imicams.ac.cn.
40. China Academic Journal e-Publishing Co., Ltd. China Network Knowledge Infrastructure. 2016; http://www.cnki.net.
41. VIP Information Co., Ltd. Chinese Scientific Journals Database. 2016; http://vip.hbdlib.cn.
42. D'Agostino RJ. Propensity score methods for bias reduction in the comparison of a treatment to a non-randomized control group. Stat Med. 1998;17:2265–81.
43. Sato T, Matsuyama Y. Marginal structural models as a tool for standardization. Epidemiology. 2003;14:680–6.
44. Witt CM, Aickin M, Cherkin D, Che CT, Elder C, Flower A, Hammerschlag R, Liu JP, Lao L, Phurrough S, Ritenbaugh C, Rubin LH, Schnyer R, Wayne PM, Withers SR, Zhao-Xiang B, Young J. Berman BM. Collaborators. Effectiveness guidance document (EGD) for Chinese medicine trials: a consensus document. Trials. 2014;15:169.
45. Yang H, Yang J, Wen Z, Zha Q, Nie G, Huang X, Zhang C, Lu A, Jiang M, Wang X. Effect of combining therapy with traditional Chinese medicine-based psychotherapy and herbal medicines in women with menopausal syndrome: a randomized controlled clinical trial. Evid Based Complement Altern Med. 2012;2012:354145.
46. Li J, Liu Z, Chen R, Hu D, Li W, Li X, Chen X, Huang B, Liao L. The quality of reports of randomized clinical trials on traditional Chinese medicine treatments: a systematic review of articles indexed in the China National Knowledge Infrastructure database from 2005 to 2012. BMC Complement Altern Med. 2014;14:362.

Chapter 4
Placebo-Controlled Trials in Acupuncture: Problems and Solutions

Stephen Birch, Terje Alraek, Kun Hyung Kim and Myeong Soo Lee

Abstract The objective of this chapter is to provide an overview of the problems and solutions of randomized placebo-controlled trials in acupuncture. Studies examining how acupuncture might work cover a broad range of physiological systems, ranging from a single biochemical pathway to the whole biological system. Needling, touch, and pressure occur before skin penetration and then surface receptors/structures are stimulated by both shallow and deeper insertions with additional receptors are further stimulated by deeper insertions. This process raises important questions about the use of penetrating and non-penetrating sham acupuncture techniques and placebo effects. In clinical research the placebo treatment must be inert, and only when the provided randomization and blinding are properly used, a trial comparing the test treatment to the placebo treatment can be said as placebo-controlled. A placebo-controlled trial is an explanatory trial since it tests the known mechanisms associated with the treatment. But in hands-on therapies like acupuncture what can constitute a valid placebo control treatment? Are there predictable mechanisms by which acupuncture works suggesting which valid placebo can be used? Are there any sham acupuncture

S. Birch (✉) · T. Alraek
Institute of Health Sciences, Kristiania University College, Oslo, Norway
e-mail: stephen.birch@kristiania.no

T. Alraek
Department of Community Medicine, Faculty of Health Sciences,
National Research Center in Complementary and Alternative Medicine (NAFKAM),
UiT The Arctic University of Norway, Tromsø, Norway
e-mail: terje.alrak@uit.no

K.H. Kim
Department of Acupuncture and Moxibustion, Korean Medicine Hospital,
Pusan National University, Yangsan, Korea
e-mail: pdchrist@gmail.com

M.S. Lee (✉)
Clinical Research Division, Korea Institute of Oriental Medicine,
Daejeon, Republic of Korea
e-mail: drmslee@gmail.com

S. Leung and H. Hu (eds.), *Evidence-based Research Methods for Chinese Medicine*, DOI 10.1007/978-981-10-2290-6_4

interventions that can constitute placebo treatments? Are they credible to be sham treatments? If they are not inert or credible, then how can we perform placebo-controlled trials on acupuncture? Are such trials possible? Many forms of sham acupuncture have been tried out in efforts to control placebo effects. In the 'real' or 'test' acupuncture the 'real' technique is applied to the 'real' acupoints. Thus, sham acupuncture involves varying the techniques of treatment and the locations of treatment. Given these two variables, three basic variations of sham acupuncture are possible. One of these could possibly act as a placebo control research model, provided that the sham techniques are clinically inert and the sites of their application are clinically inert. The other two models act to compare either treatment sites or treatment techniques. In the latter two models placebo can be held equal between treatment groups, but these models are not capable of acting as placebo-controlled trials. The second and third sham models are often used inadvertently as though they were capable of answering the same question as the first or were placebo-controlled clinical trials like the first. This chapter will give an overview on the current status and problems of placebo-controlled trials in acupuncture trials and suggest possible solutions. We can summarize the evidence: so far no sham acupuncture techniques are inert; they are also clinically effective; and no placebo-controlled trials of acupuncture have ever been performed. Given the evidence, we propose to stop performing sham acupuncture studies since they cannot achieve control for placebo effects. We propose a two-pronged approach to address the issues of mechanisms of action and effectiveness.

Keywords Acupuncture · Placebo · Sham · Clinical trial · Acupoint

4.1 Introduction

The act of inserting needles for the practice of acupuncture can trigger multiple pathways, many of which are predictable from knowledge of biology since the living organism has multiple sensory systems for interacting with the environment and responding to its challenges. Biological effects can occur as a result of touch and pressure [26, 27, 41, 48, 60, 66, 85], pricking and other non-insertion methods [41, 65], skin penetration (shallow insertion) [3, 39, 40, 57, 78, 87], stimulation of underlying structures (deeper insertion) and manipulation of the needle (rotation, lifting-thrusting) [30, 31, 45, 68, 71, 87]. Many of these pathways have already been demonstrated with regards to acupuncture needling [6, 14–16, 20, 30, 31, 37, 68, 71, 87, 88] and can involve analgesic [14, 30, 31, 68, 87], anti-inflammatory [61, 89], micro-circulatory [37, 39], circulatory [53, 82], immunologic [1, 62, 86], autonomic [49, 51, 64, 78] and modulation of the somatosensory system [5, 63] effects. Brain imaging studies have demonstrated different responses with both different needling techniques and different locations of the needling [34, 36, 70], suggesting a degree of specificity of effects supported by biological analysis of tissue structures and pathways involved [46, 87]. Since the practice of acupuncture involves application of touch, pressure and usually pricking, shallow and deep insertion and with various needle manipulations, then any of the above effects can occur with acupuncture needling, regardless of where and how the needling is done. Studies examining the neurological effects of needling have found that sham acupuncture techniques activate different pathways than the test acupuncture techniques [3, 20, 41, 50, 57, 64], suggesting that they are not inert. Hence, it is also important to examine whether there is evidence that they are also clinically active and especially effective. A sham technique that is physiologically active may still be relevant in efforts to control for placebo effects even if it is not clinically relevant/active. The above physiological effects/evidence raises important questions for the implementation of the studies that attempt to control for placebo effects in acupuncture. A placebo intervention is supposed to be physiologically inert; however, they must be credible for the exposed participants How might one apply a placebo needling technique that can avoid all of the above effects so that it is inert, and can thus act as a placebo control intervention for clinical trials of acupuncture? If it is not possible to avoid some of these physiological effects, are they clinically active? Given the evidence of physiological activity among sham techniques, how does one implement and interpret clinical trials?

4.2 Acupuncture and Sham Acupuncture

Acupuncture involves the use of needles applied to specific acupoints. These have locations that have been described relative to anatomical structures and are usually assumed to be fixed relative to those structures. A common form of needling since the 1950s employs a method whereby needles are inserted into the acupoints to specified depths for each acupoint and then manipulated until certain sensations called 'deqi' are obtained (soreness, aching, distension, heaviness, numbness or tingling) [8, 17, 25]. Textbooks routinely state that if these sensations are not obtained with needling, then the treatment will not be effective [17, 44]. Since the first descriptions of this deqi in Western publications in the early 1970s, researchers have tested acupuncture in controlled trials that attempt to control for placebo effects by varying the locations of the needling and the techniques of needling using what has been called 'sham acupuncture' [10]. In particular, during the last 30 years needling techniques have been used to avoid producing the deqi sensations. Some review papers have catalogued the types of sham acupuncture techniques that can be found in acupuncture trials and the clinical questions that they can answer [9, 23]. Since 1983, clinical trials started using shallow needle insertion (2–3 mm) with no manipulation [21, 32, 33, 80] in an effort to avoid the deqi sensations and serve the role of a placebo control. In the late 1990s, stage dagger-like needles that do not penetrate the skin emerged, first the Streitberger needle [74], then the Park needle [67] and more recently the Japanese sham needle from Takakura [77] and a Chinese variant [52]. While these non-penetrating sham techniques do not penetrate the skin, they do apply pressure and some give pricking and deqi sensations [69, 76]. The two methods of shallow insertion without needle manipulation and non-penetrating sham needling have become the two most common forms of sham acupuncture and are often thought to produce only placebo effects. Some research groups have used sham TENS [24] or sham laser [35] as control treatment for acupuncture. Since these sham treatments do not match the appearance of acupuncture, it has been suggested that they are better avoided in placebo-controlled studies [47] and have been criticized as 'fatally-flawed' for acupuncture studies [79]. These different sham needling techniques have been verified with regards to their credibility for clinical trials of acupuncture usually by testing whether patients could tell which needling method they received [76, 81]. An equally important sub-study to validate the sham procedures is to examine whether the techniques are inert or not and if not, to develop procedures capable of dealing with the unasked for effects by eliminating or controlling for them [11, 59]. We know of very few studies that have attempted to do this [4, 7]. We have not found any studies that have demonstrated that the techniques are inert, rather we have found authors acknowledging that the techniques are not inert [2, 27, 55, 56, 83]. Since there are both physiological evidence and clinically informed opinions that they are not inert, it is also important to understand whether these physiological effects can produce clinically relevant changes.

4.3 Sham Procedures

Given the two variables of location of needling and technique of needling there are three basic variations of sham acupuncture (Table 4.1).

The sham type 3 clinical trial allows us to examine the clinical effectiveness of the proposed sham techniques, *while holding placebo equal between the two*

Table 4.1 Acupuncture-sham acupuncture test components, sham variations and their uses

	Technique	Acupoints	Potential uses
'Real' acupuncture	Real (RT)	Real (RAP)	The test treatment
Sham acupuncture-1	Sham (ST)	Sham (non) (SAP)	The sham treatment—potentially capable of acting as a placebo treatment
Sham acupuncture-2	Same as real (RT)	Sham (SAP)	Tests relative effects of point location[a]
Sham acupuncture-3	Sham (ST)	Same as real (RAP)	Tests relative effects of needle techniques[a]

[a]These two sham models are NOT tests of acupuncture per se, rather they are tests of the relative effects of the places of needling or the techniques of needling [10, 84]. Yet they are routinely used as though they were sham acupuncture-1 type studies, as valid tests of acupuncture and then confused further when said to be placebo treatments [72, 75]. These studies by their nature cannot control for placebo effects [12, 13], they are similar to studies of a drug at different dose levels or comparison of different drug mixes

treatment groups. When the sham treatment technique is more effective than the test treatment technique, it indicates that the sham technique is clinically effective. Similarly, if the sham technique is as effective as the test treatment technique for a specific condition and systematic reviews of acupuncture for that technique show that acupuncture is an effective treatment, this too can indicate that the sham technique can be clinically effective. Thus in order to answer the question of whether sham type 1 trials are able to control for placebo effects, we can examine sham type 3 trials to understand the effect and role of the sham techniques themselves.

The following clinical trials illustrate that the non-penetrating or shallow needling sham technique can be more effective than normal needling for certain conditions or as effective as normal needling in conditions for which evidence shows normal needling works [22, 54, 72, 73, 75]. Other clinical trials also demonstrate that shallow needling can be more effective than a touch only sham needling [28, 42, 43]. We thus have evidence that both the shallow insertion and the non-penetrating sham are clinically effective techniques.

4.4 Implications of the Physiologically Active and Clinically Effective Sham Acupuncture Technique

There is clear evidence that the more commonly used sham techniques of shallow insertion 'minimal acupuncture' and non-penetrating sham (stage dagger needles) are both physiologically active and clinically effective techniques, independent of placebo effects. The likely explanation for this is that both procedures involve touch with pressure and pricking, and the former also involves shallow insertion. This makes these sham procedures unsuitable for use as control treatments for placebo control trials of acupuncture. Rather studies that use these sham procedures are instead a form of dose comparison trials and thus 'pragmatic trials' that allow for investigation of the different types of stimulation needed to reduce the symptoms in question.

The fact that both procedures utilize some of the pathways involved in the theoretically proscribed treatment also introduces further complications. De Craen and colleagues have demonstrated that a sham treatment that is inadvertently active rather than inert and involves the same pathways as the test treatment creates bias against the test treatment [19]. In line with this recent authors have suggested that sham acupuncture procedures introduce a risk of bias against acupuncture by underestimating the effects of treatment [2, 58]. The uncovering of these issues has led an international expert group to suggest that sham acupuncture procedures to be discontinued at least in clinical trials [46].

4.5 Recommendations

We cannot see how it is possible to conduct a placebo-controlled clinical trial of acupuncture. None of the sham techniques that have been developed and used are capable of acting as placebo treatments. Further, independent of placebo effects they will instead trigger some of the pathways of action by which acupuncture works, thereby underestimating the effects of acupuncture and introducing a risk of bias against acupuncture. We agree with Langevin and colleagues that it could still be helpful outside of clinical trials to use some sham acupuncture procedures in physiological acupuncture research [46]. We feel that the proposals of Hyland [38] and Langevin et al. [46] should be developed for future research on acupuncture.

The explanatory or placebo-controlled trial is fundamentally a clinical test of a known mechanism of a therapy. We have seen that acupuncture effects can involve multiple pathways of action simultaneously. The specific components of these pathways will vary considerably according to location of needling and manner of needling. This makes the pathways of action that are to be controlled for in trials that attempt to control for placebo effects unpredictable and unknown. Placebo-controlled trials are simply not achievable for acupuncture studies, at least at this time, *thus sham acupuncture techniques should not be used in clinical trials of acupuncture*.

We feel that the inherent complexity and variability of how acupuncture can work is better studied by taking advantage of developments in the field of systems biology [18, 29] and OMICS [16]. With more careful attention to the dynamics of how the different pathways work and interact, gradually a more clear picture of acupuncture should emerge.

Since placebo effects cannot be controlled for in a head to head comparison of acupuncture and placebo treatment (the explanatory trial), sham acupuncture trials should not be used. Instead pragmatic trials should be used, where the control treatment is either an established standard therapy or when relevant a no-treatment group should be added. These pragmatic trials should be used alongside with physiological studies in carefully orchestrated ways for exploration of the hypothesized or established mechanisms of clinical acupuncture.

References

1. Aguiar DN, Silva MM, Parreira WV, et al. Electroacupuncture at the ST36 acupoint increases interleukin-4 responsiveness in macrophages, generation of alternatively activated macrophages and susceptibility to *Leishmania* major infection. Chin Med. 2012;7:17.
2. Appleyard I, Lundeberg T, Robinson N. Should systematic reviews assess the risk of bias from sham–placebo acupuncture control procedures? Eur J Integr Med. 2014;6:234–43.
3. Asghar AU, Green G, Lythgoe MF, et al. Acupuncture needling sensation: the neural correlates of deqi using fMRI. Brain Res. 2010;1315:111–8.
4. Avants SK, Margolin A, Holford TR, et al. A randomized controlled trial of auricular acupuncture for cocaine dependence. Arch Intern Med. 2000;160:2305–12.

5. Baeumler PI, Fleckenstein J, Takayama S, et al. Effects of acupuncture on sensory perception: a systematic review and meta-analysis. PLoS ONE. 2014;9:e113731.
6. Bai L, Lao L. Neurobiological foundations of acupuncture: the relevance and future prospect based on neuroimaging evidence. Evid Based Complement Alternat Med. 2013;2013:812568.
7. Birch S, Jamison RN. Controlled trial of Japanese acupuncture for chronic myofascial neck pain: assessment of specific and nonspecific effects of treatment. Clin J Pain. 1998;14:248–55.
8. Birch S, Felt R. Understanding acupuncture. Edinburgh: Churchill Livingstone; 1999.
9. Birch S. Overview of models used in controlled acupuncture studies and thoughts about questions answerable by each. Clin Acupunct Oriental Med. 2002;3:207–17.
10. Birch S, Hammerschlag R, Trinh K, et al. The non-specific effects of acupuncture treatment: when and how to control for them. Clin Acupunct Oriental Med. 2002;3:20–5.
11. Birch S. Clinical research on acupuncture. Part 2. Controlled clinical trials, an overview of their methods. J Altern Complement Med. 2004;10:481–98.
12. Birch S. Sham acupuncture is not a placebo-implications and problems in research. JAM. 2012;2:5–9.
13. Birch S. Historical and clinical perspectives on de qi: exposing limitations in the scientific study of de qi. J Altern Complement Med. 2015;21:1–7.
14. Bowsher D. Mechanisms of acupuncture. In: Filshie J, White A, editors. Medical acupuncture. Edinburgh: Churchill Livingstone; 1998. p. 69–83.
15. Chae Y, Chang DS, Lee SH, et al. Inserting needles into the body: a meta-analysis of brain activity associated with acupuncture needle stimulation. J Pain. 2013;14:215–22.
16. Chen R, Mias GI, Li-Pook-Than J, et al. Personal omics profiling reveals dynamic molecular and medical phenotypes. Cell. 2012; 148(6):1293–1307.
17. Cheng XN. Chinese acupuncture and moxibustion. Beijing: Foreign Languages Press; 1987.
18. Chuang HY, Hofree M, Ideker T. A decade of systems biology. Annu Rev Cell Dev Biol. 2010;26:721–44.
19. De Craen AJ, Tijssen JG, Kleijnen J. Is there a need to control the placebo in placebo controlled trials? Heart. 1997;77:95–6.
20. Dhond RP, Kettner N, Napadow V. Neuroimaging acupuncture effects in the human brain. J Altern Complement Med. 2007;13:603–16.
21. Dhond RP, Yeh C, Park K, et al. Acupuncture modulates resting state connectivity in default and sensorimotor brain networks. Pain. 2008;136:407–18.
22. Dieterle S, Li C, Greb R, et al. A prospective randomized placebo-controlled study of the effect of acupuncture in infertile patients with severe oligoasthenozoospermia. Fertil Steril. 2009;92:1340–3.
23. Dincer F, Linde K. Sham interventions in randomized clinical trials of acupuncture—a review. Complement Ther Med. 2003;11:235–42.
24. Dowson DI, Lewith GT, Machin D. The effects of acupuncture versus placebo in the treatment of headache. Pain. 1985;21:35–42.
25. Ellis A, Wiseman N, Boss K. Fundamentals of Chinese acupuncture. Brookline: Paradigm Publications; 1991.
26. Fields T. Touch therapy. London: Churchill Livingstone; 2000.
27. Fregni F, Imamura M, Chien HF, et al. Challenges and recommendations for placebo controls in randomized trials in physical and rehabilitation medicine: a report of the international placebo symposium working group. Am J Phys Med Rehabil. 2010;89:160–72.
28. Furuya E, Nayuki T, Yakame M, et al. The effects of press tack needle treatment on upper back muscle stiffness—comparative study using sham needle. JAM. 2009;1:12–21.
29. Gonzalez-Angulo AM, Hennessy BT, Mills GB. Future of personalized medicine in oncology: a systems biology approach. J Clin Oncol. 2010;28:2777–83.
30. Han JS. Physiology of acupuncture: a review of thirty years of research. J Altern Complement Med. 1997;3:S1.
31. Han JS. Acupuncture analgesia: areas of consensus and controversy. Pain. 2011;152:S41–8.

32. Hansen PE, Hansen JH. Acupuncture treatment of chronic facial pain—a controlled cross-over trial. Headache. 1983;23:66–9.
33. Hansen PE, Hansen JH. Acupuncture treatment of chronic tension headache—a controlled cross-over trial. Cephalalgia. 1985;5:137–42.
34. Harris RE, Zubieta JK, Scott DJ, et al. Traditional Chinese acupuncture and placebo (sham) acupuncture are differentiated by their effects on mu-opioid receptors (MORs). Neuroimage. 2009;47:1077–85.
35. Hinman RS, McCrory P, Pirotta M, et al. Acupuncture for chronic knee pain: a randomized clinical trial. JAMA. 2014;312:1313–22.
36. Huang T, Wang RH, Zhang WB, et al. The influence of different methods of acupuncture on skin surface perfusion. J Tradit Chin Med. 2012;32:40–4.
37. Huang W, Pach D, Napadow V, et al. Characterizing acupuncture stimuli using brain imaging with FMRI—a systematic review and meta-analysis of the literature. PLoS ONE. 2012;7: e32960.
38. Hyland ME. Methodology for the scientific evaluation of complementary and alternative medicine. Complement Ther Med. 2003;11:146–53.
39. Itaya K, Manaka Y, Ohkubo C, et al. Effects of acupuncture needle application upon cutaneous microcirculation of rabbit ear lobe. Acupunct Electrother Res. 1987;12:45–51.
40. Jung WS, Park SU, Park JM, et al. Changes in SPECT cerebral blood flow following Japanese style, superficial acupuncture at LI-4 and LI-11 in healthy volunteers. J Altern Complement Med. 2011;17:357–62.
41. Kawakita K, Shinbara H, Imai K, et al. How do acupuncture and moxibustion act? Focusing on the progress in Japanese acupuncture research. J Pharmacol Sci. 2006;100:443–59.
42. Kim YS, Lee SH, Jung WS, et al. Intradermal acupuncture on shen-men and nei-kuan acupoints in patients with insomnia after stroke. Am J Chin Med. 2004;32:771–8.
43. Kotani N, Hashimoto H, Sato Y, et al. Preoperative intradermal acupuncture reduces postoperative pain, nausea and vomiting, analgesic requirement, and sympathoadrenal responses. Anesthesiology. 2001;95:349–56.
44. Lai XS, Tong Z. A study on the classification and the 'catching' of the 'arrived qi' in acupuncture. J Tradit Chin Med. 2010;30:3–8.
45. Langevin HM, Churchill DL, Wu J, et al. Evidence of connective tissue involvement in acupuncture. FASEB J. 2002;16:872–4.
46. Langevin HM, Wayne PM, Macpherson H, et al. Paradoxes in acupuncture research: strategies for moving forward. Evid Based Complement Alternat Med. 2011;2011:180805.
47. Lao L, Ezzo J, Berman BM, et al. Assessing clinical efficacy of acupuncture: considerations for designing future acupuncture trials. In: Stux G, Hammerschlag R, editors. Clinical acupuncture: scientific basis. Berlin: Springer; 2000. p. 187–209.
48. Leder D, Krucoff MW. The touch that heals: the uses and meanings of touch in the clinical encounter. J Altern Complement Med. 2008;14:321–7.
49. Lee MHM, Ernst M. Clinical research observations on acupuncture analgesia and thermography. In: Stux G, Pomeranz B, editors. Scientific bases of acupuncture. Berlin: Springerp; 1988. p. 157–175.
50. Lewith G, Barlow F, Eyles C, et al. The context and meaning of placebos for complementary medicine. Forsch Komplementmed. 2009;16:404–12.
51. Li QQ, Shi GX, Xu Q, et al. Acupuncture effect and central autonomic regulation. Evid Based Complement Alternat Med. 2013;2013:267959.
52. Liu B, Xu H, Ma R, et al. Effect of blinding with a new pragmatic placebo needle: a randomized controlled crossover study. Medicine (Baltimore). 2014;93:e200.
53. Longhurst J. Acupuncture's cardiovascular actions: a mechanistic perspective. Med Acupunct. 2013;25:101–13.
54. Lund I, Lundeberg T, Lonnberg L, et al. Decrease of pregnant women's pelvic pain after acupuncture: a randomized controlled single-blind study. Acta Obstet Gynecol Scand. 2006;85:12–9.

55. Lund I, Naslund J, Lundeberg T. Minimal acupuncture is not a valid placebo control in randomised controlled trials of acupuncture: a physiologist's perspective. Chin Med. 2009;4:1.
56. Lundeberg T, Lund I, Sing A, et al. Is placebo acupuncture what it is intended to be? Evid Based Complement Alternat Med. 2011;2011:932407.
57. MacPherson H, Green G, Nevado A, et al. Brain imaging of acupuncture: comparing superficial with deep needling. Neurosci Lett. 2008;434:144–9.
58. MacPherson H, Vertosick E, Lewith G, et al. Influence of control group on effect size in trials of acupuncture for chronic pain: a secondary analysis of an individual patient data meta-analysis. PLoS ONE. 2014;9:e93739.
59. Margolin A, Avants SK, Kleber HD. Rationale and design of the cocaine alternative treatments study (CATS): a randomized, controlled trial of acupuncture. J Altern Complement Med. 1998;4:405–18.
60. McCraty R, Atkinson M, Tomasino D, et al. The electricity of touch: detection and measurement of cardiac energy exchange between people. In: Pribram KH, editor. Brain and values: is a biological science of values possible? New Jergey: Lawrence Erlbaum Associates, Inc.; 1998. p. 359–79.
61. McDonald JL, Cripps AW, Smith PK, et al. The anti-inflammatory effects of acupuncture and their relevance to allergic rhinitis: a narrative review and proposed model. Evid Based Complement Alternat Med. 2013;2013:591796.
62. Mori H, Nishijo K, Kawamura H, et al. Unique immunomodulation by electro-acupuncture in humans possibly via stimulation of the autonomic nervous system. Neurosci Lett. 2002;320:21–4.
63. Napadow V, Dhond RP, Kim J, et al. Brain encoding of acupuncture sensation–coupling on-line rating with fMRI. Neuroimage. 2009;47:1055–65.
64. Nishijo K, Mori H, Yosikawa K, et al. Decreased heart rate by acupuncture stimulation in humans via facilitation of cardiac vagal activity and suppression of cardiac sympathetic nerve. Neurosci Lett. 1997;227:165–8.
65. O'Brien KA, Birch S, Abbas E, et al. Traditional East Asian medical pulse diagnosis: a preliminary physiologic investigation. J Altern Complement Med. 2013;19:793–8.
66. Olausson H, Lamarre Y, Backlund H, et al. Unmyelinated tactile afferents signal touch and project to insular cortex. Nat Neurosci. 2002;5:900–4.
67. Park J, White A, Lee H, et al. Development of a new sham needle. Acupunct Med. 1999;17:110–2.
68. Pomeranz B, Berman B. Scientific basis of acupuncture. In: Stux G, Berman B, Pomeranz B, editors. Basics of acupuncture. Berlin: Springer; 2003. p. 1–86.
69. Salih N, Baumler PI, Simang M, et al. Deqi sensations without cutaneous sensory input: results of an RCT. BMC Complement Altern Med. 2010;10:81.
70. Shan Y, Wang ZQ, Zhao ZL, et al. An FMRI study of neuronal specificity in acupuncture: the multiacupoint siguan and its sham point. Evid Based Complement Alternat Med. 2014;2014:103491.
71. Shang C. Prospective tests on biological models of acupuncture. Evid Based Complement Alternat Med. 2009;6:31–9.
72. So EW, Ng EH, Wong YY, et al. A randomized double blind comparison of real and placebo acupuncture in IVF treatment. Hum Reprod. 2009;24:341–8.
73. So EW, Ng EH, Wong YY, et al. Acupuncture for frozen-thawed embryo transfer cycles: a double-blind randomized controlled trial. Reprod Biomed Online. 2010;20:814–21.
74. Streitberger K, Kleinhenz J. Introducing a placebo needle into acupuncture research. Lancet. 1998;352:364–5.
75. Streitberger K, Friedrich-Rust M, Bardenheuer H, et al. Effect of acupuncture compared with placebo-acupuncture at P6 as additional antiemetic prophylaxis in high-dose chemotherapy and autologous peripheral blood stem cell transplantation: a randomized controlled single-blind trial. Clin Cancer Res. 2003;9:2538–44.
76. Takakura N, Yajima H. A placebo acupuncture needle with potential for double blinding—a validation study. Acupunct Med. 2008;26:224–30.

77. Takakura N, Takayama M, Kawase A, et al. Tapping-in method (skin penetration technique) with a placebo needle for double-blind acupuncture trials. J Altern Complement Med. 2013;19:308–12.
78. Tanaka TH, Leisman G, Nishijo K. The physiological responses induced by superficial acupuncture: a comparative study of acupuncture stimulation during exhalation phase and continuous stimulation. Int J Neurosci. 1997;90:45–58.
79. ter Riet G, Kleijnen J, Knipschild P. Acupuncture and chronic pain: a criteria-based meta-analysis. J Clin Epidemiol. 1990;43:1191–9.
80. Vincent CA. A controlled trial of the treatment of migraine by acupuncture. Clin J Pain. 1989;5:305–12.
81. Vincent CA. Credibility assessment in trials of acupuncture. Complement Med Res. 1990;4:8–11.
82. Watanabe M, Takayama S, Yamamoto Y, et al. Haemodynamic changes in the superior mesenteric artery induced by acupuncture stimulation on the lower limbs. Evid Based Complement Alternat Med. 2012;2012:908546.
83. White A. Acupuncture research methodology. In: Lewith G, Jonas WB, Walach H, editors. Clinical research in complementary therapies. Edinburgh: Churchill Livingstone; 2002. p. 307–23.
84. White AR, Filshie J, Cummings TM, et al. Clinical trials of acupuncture: consensus recommendations for optimal treatment, sham controls and blinding. Complement Ther Med. 2001;9:237–45.
85. Witzel T, Napadow V, Kettner NW, et al. Differences in cortical response to acupressure and electroacupuncture stimuli. BMC Neurosci. 2011;12:73.
86. Yamaguchi N, Takahashi T, Sakuma M, et al. Acupuncture regulates leukocyte subpopulations in human peripheral blood. Evid Based Complement Alternat Med. 2007;4:447–53.
87. Zhang ZJ, Wang XM, McAlonan GM. Neural acupuncture unit: a new concept for interpreting effects and mechanisms of acupuncture. Evid Based Complement Alternat Med. 2012;2012:429412.
88. Zhao ZQ. Neural mechanism underlying acupuncture analgesia. Prog Neurobiol. 2008;85:355–75.
89. Zijlstra FJ, van den Berg-de Lange I, Huygen FJ, et al. Anti-inflammatory actions of acupuncture. Mediators Inflamm. 2003;12:59–69.

Chapter 5
Qualitative Interview for Chinese Medicine Research: Challenges and Prospects

Hao Hu, Jian Li and Hong Chen

Abstract This chapter aims at initiating discussions about how to use qualitative interviewing for Chinese medicine research. Through examining a case of practical application of this approach, it has identified three main challenges arising therefrom, viz., (1) challenge of avoiding cultural bias in sampling; (2) challenge of designing an effective interview, including the questioning techniques and (3) challenge of developing concepts and constructs that are germane to such in-depth interviews. It also provides suggestions for future qualitative study of Chinese medicine with regard to: (1) applying a strategy of comparative research; (2) developing a well-prepared interview protocol and (3) balancing views of Chinese medicine and Western medicine in data analysis.

Keywords Qualitative interview · Chinese medicine · Qualitative study · Community pharmacy · Pharmacy practice

5.1 Introduction

Research in Chinese medicine has attracted increasing attention in recent years from both within China and abroad. Apart from conducting lab experiment studies, researchers are constantly encouraged (even required) to apply qualitative methods to studying important topics related to Chinese medicine. However, they are

H. Hu (✉) · H. Chen
State Key Laboratory of Quality Research in Chinese Medicine,
Institute of Chinese Medical Sciences, University of Macau, Macau, China
e-mail: haohu@umac.mo

H. Chen
e-mail: april_chen@163.com

J. Li
Faculty of Arts and Humanities, University of Macau, Macau, China
e-mail: jamesli@umac.mo

S. Leung and H. Hu (eds.), *Evidence-based Research Methods for Chinese Medicine*, DOI 10.1007/978-981-10-2290-6_5

generally reluctant to do so because they have received their academic training mostly in natural science. Their main issue can be expressed in this question: *Why should qualitative approach be called for in Chinese medicine research?* Or *what kind of role could qualitative method actually play in Chinese medicine research?*

To address the question above, the key seems to be a shift in perspective from the researcher's to the consumer's (that of patients, doctors and others). For the latter, their personal concerns about Chinese medicine tend to focus on: *Why should I choose Chinese medicine? What Chinese medicine could treat my disease or benefit my health? How should I take Chinese medicine properly? How should I manage (regulate) Chinese medicine clinically?* These questions could well lead to significant research ground for the researchers' new endeavours.

To treat these potential topics for research, qualitative methods have their unique strengths. Qualitative methods emphasize 'meaning' of social phenomena as experienced by people in their natural setting [1, 2]. Rather than simple description of emotional and experiential phenomena, qualitative methods provide chance to understand the underlying 'how' and 'why' [3, 4].

Qualitative interview as one of the most commonly used methods in social sciences has its distinctive value in exploring the interviewee's 'meaning' through interactions between an interviewer and an interviewee [5]. Thus, regarded as an effective instrument, qualitative interview is expected to be actively applied in modern Chinese medicine research. In reality, however, this method is hardly employed as such in spite of its special function, a telltale indication that methodological challenges may have deterred the researchers in the field from using it.

Situated in this context, this chapter aims to provide some initial discussions about how to apply qualitative interviewing in studying Chinese medicine using our own example of a case study, focusing on the sampling process as well as the challenges we met. We will first review the general designing features of qualitative interview in research; then, we will report on a research case of our own using qualitative interview that was meant to elicit consumers' opinions about Chinese patent medicine versus Westernmedicine dispensed over the counter of community pharmacies. Next, we will discuss the main challenges of applying qualitative interview method to studying Chinese medicine and offer some suggestions for prospective qualitative interviews in this field; and finally, some conclusive remarks.

5.2 General Design of Qualitative Interview Research

Following the general guidelines on qualitative research, qualitative interview is so designed as to make sure the three key parameters are clearly defined: sampling, interview protocol and data analysis.

5.2.1 *Sampling for Qualitative Interview*

Qualitative interview does not follow the random sampling approach that is widely applied in quantitative research. On the contrary, qualitative interview generally adopts a purposeful sampling approach. Qualitative purposeful sampling means that researcher decide on their sample according to the research objectives, which may differentiate between types of cases as being typical, unusual, critical, politically important, etc. [6]. In particular, there is a general consensus that theoretical sampling is also a kind of purposeful sampling even though it is theory-driven to some extent [7]. In fact, it can be said that all sampling is purposeful in qualitative research.

More recently, qualitative researchers argue for 'information power' generated in a well-planned sampling process. In their words, for qualitative interview sampling, 5 factors need to be taken into account: (1) the aim of the study; (2) sample specificity; (3) use of established theory; (4) quality of dialogue and (5) analysis strategy. Therefore, it is incumbent upon researchers to estimate their research project systematically in sampling decision-making [8].

5.2.2 *Interview Protocol Development*

For researchers, there are three types of interviews with their choice: structured, semi-structured; and depth [5]. For any of these interview types, researchers must prepare interview protocol for their study. They need to plan carefully what questions they should ask, how to ask, and how to interact with the responses of their study participants in real time. More importantly, researchers need to clarify their own research objective and strategy in developing the interview protocol, for example, they can ask questions on different subjects for whatever details about respondents' lives, circumstances, experiences, knowledge, belief, thoughts, feelings and behaviours. Currently, interview protocol is required for ethics evaluation by most universities around the world.

5.2.3 *Data Analysis in Qualitative Interviewing*

For data analysis from qualitative interviews, several approaches have been developed, including thematic approach, framework approach, etc. Compared with framework approach [9], the former deserves more attention. Thematic approach is designed to develop key themes and identify the relationships among themes. The application of this approach generally follows the six steps [10]:

(1) Familiarizing yourself with your data,
(2) Generating initial codes,

(3) Searching for themes,
(4) Reviewing themes,
(5) Defining and naming themes and
(6) Producing the report.

By applying thematic approach, researchers focus not just on finding out the key themes from the interview data but also examining how the themes are interconnected. In this capacity, thematic approach is used to develop models or schemas, even taxonomies or classifications, to demonstrate the relationships among themes [11]. As such, thematic approach could be used to target theory development [12].

5.3 An Example of Doing Chinese Medicine Research Using Qualitative Interview Method

5.3.1 Research Objective

The main objective of this study is to explore consumers' opinions about Chinese patent medicine versus Western medicine purchased at community pharmacies. From the perspective of pharmaceutical care, it aims specifically at understanding the characteristics of customer care for consumers of Chinese patent medicine and Western medicine in comparison.

5.3.2 Method

5.3.2.1 Research Approach and Setting

Qualitative interview was chosen as research approach for this study. As ideas about Chinese patent medicine and Western medicine are highly related to personal mindset as regards health and drugs, qualitative interview promises to be the appropriate means to investigate the attitude and perceptions of individual consumers. The whole project was approved by the Ethics Committee at University of Macau.

The subject of this interview study is defined as residents of the City Proper Yinchuan which is composed of Xingqing, Jinfeng and Xixia Districts, who were over 20 years of age, speaking Mandarin, and purchased OTC drugs at the local pharmacies within the last 6 months. There was no differentiation made with regard to the type and scale of the community pharmacies at which they shopped. Pedestrians were randomly picked for an invitation to our interview at three loci in each of the three city districts of Yinchuan, who were to become the interviewees if they accepted our interview questions as well as the introduction of our research purpose. No target sample size was set for this research; it was deemed adequate as soon as the saturation of data was reached.

5.3.2.2 Data Collection

An interview protocol was prepared for study. The protocol was designed to include the explanatory notes and open-ended questions. It was drawn up in a test version at first, which was used in mock-up interviews that involved 3 physicians and pharmacists working in the pharmaceutical business, as well as 7 regular consumers of the drugs. Next, part of the wording was revised according to the result of the trial run and the feedback received. Once again the improved version was put on a feasibility test in interviews with 10 randomly picked regular consumers, before it was settled for the final version of the interview protocol.

The questions for interviews mainly consist of two parts: general demographic information of the interviewee, and their ideas about Chinese patent medicine versus Western medicine (see Table 5.1).

According to the status quo of community pharmacies in China, the pharmacists being referred to in this study include both pharmacists and licensed pharmacists, who are ranked by junior titles (pharmacist or pharmacist of TCM), intermediate titles (competent pharmacist or supervisor of Chinese medicine) and senior titles (deputy director pharmacist and director pharmacist; deputy director of Chinese medicine and director of Chinese medicine).

The interviews started on January 28th, 2015 and ended March 24th, lasting 55 days. The semi-structured interview was carried out vis-a-vis, with each anonymous respondent taking up 15 min or so. Questions were asked item by item in the planned order to the consumer in the interview. The conversation was taped

Table 5.1 Main interview questions

A. *General demographic information*
• Gender
• Age
• Education
• Occupation
B. *Consumer idea about Chinese patent medicine versus Western medicine*
(1) For OTC drugs, do you prefer to purchase Chinese patent drug or Western medicine? Why?
(2) Of which medicine, Chinese or western, are you more likely to need a community pharmacist's help for the purchase? What kind of information seems to cause you more confusion?
(3) Do you have difficulty understanding the instruction for a Chinese patent drug or that for Western medicine, such as indications, contraindications, warnings and precautions or interactions with other drugs?

by mutual consent and recorded verbatim in Microsoft Excel 2011 files. Each interview went on as long as there was no more relevant new information to emerge.

5.3.2.3 Data Analysis

The results of the interviews were examined with the invalid cases eliminated. The consumers' opinions were summarized and salient points highlighted. Those that were eliminated should meet the criteria that either the interview was deemed uncompleted for any reason, or it contradicts itself significantly as there was a wide discrepancy found between the answers provided at the beginning of the interview and the later ones. Thematic analysis was adopted to process the data for this study. By perusing the data file many times over to get conversant with the views of the respondents, we were able to mark off the reoccurring themes and new themes, and find out the linkages between them.

5.3.3 Results: Chinese Patent Medicine Versus Western Medicine

It shows that 57 of our interviewees claimed that they were inclined to acquire Chinese patent medicine, whereas 31 tended to purchase Western medicine. We followed up on this division of choice to explore the differentiation of purchasing preference for either Chinese patent medicine or Western medicine among the regular consumers.

5.3.3.1 Purchase Predisposition

For the majority of the consumers of non-prescription drugs, the inclination to stay in favour of Chinese patent medicine is caused by the belief that it is safer than Western medicine. As mentioned by our interviewees:

> "… [I] prefer Chinese patent medicine, [which has] little side effects …" (27, male, bachelor's degree)
>
> "… [regarding] Chinese patent medicine … I don't feel much of its side effects …" (29, male, junior college graduate)
>
> "… [regarding] Chinese patent medicine … it is mild and has minimal side effects …" (37, male, bachelor's degree)
>
> "… [compared with] Chinese patent medicine … Western medicine has lots more harmful aftereffects …" (32, female, junior college graduate)

Some consumers believe that Western medicine only treats the symptoms but not effect a permanent cure; therefore, they opt for Chinese patent medicine. As described by one interviewee:

> "… [regarding Chinese patent medicine] … [it]has less side effects, whereas western medicine offers only temporary solution not a cure to the root cause…" (54, female, junior high school graduate)

Others, influenced by the Chinese medicine culture, hold that Chinese patent medicine offer more effective solutions to curing the intrinsic problems, hence their preference for it.

> "… [regarding] Chinese patent medicine … [I] didn't give much thought … got used to it … " (27, female, bachelor's degree)

> "… [regarding] Chinese patent medicine … I believe in Chinese medicine more … " (23, female, bachelor's degree)

> "… [regarding] Chinese patent medicine … it has higher credibility …" (45, female, junior college graduate)

> "… [regarding] Chinese patent medicine … I find it more effective, having few side effects, and recuperating as well …" (27, male, bachelor's degree)

Those who tend to buy Western medicine are generally driven by their demand for quick cures, as they share the unspoken belief that Chinese patent medicine is incapable of catering for what they need.

> "… [regarding] western medicine … it offers a quick cure …" (25, female, master's degree)

> "… [regarding] western medicine … it has quicker curative effect, while Chinese medicine seems much milder …" (25, male, master's degree)

Most of the pro-western medicine consumers are predisposed to taking Western medicine for treatment as a consequence of receiving their doctors' prescriptions for Western medication in most of their hospital experiences. As described by one interviewee:

> "… [regarding] western medicine … like regular prescriptions by doctors, so I am used to it …" (64, male, elementary schooling)

That some lean towards choosing Western medicine is due to the fact that recent years saw, on the one hand, those time-honoured well-known brands of Western medicine upholding their good name for curative power but at minimal cost; and an incessant price climb of Chinese patent medicine on the other hand. As described by one interviewee:

> "… [regarding] western medicine … unlike Chinese patent medicine that shows no immediate effect but fairly expensive …" (28, female, bachelor's degree)

The disadvantages of the dosage form of Chinese patent medicine, i.e., lack of handiness and oral rejection of its taste, also give rise to preference for Western medicine among those consumers. Some interviewees mentioned:

"… [compared with] western medicine … because Chinese patent medicine is generally bitter in taste …" (48, female, senior high school graduate)

"… [to take] western medicine … it is good for quick swallow …" (35, male, junior college graduate)

Such consumers are found in favour of Chinese–Western medicine compound recipe, acknowledging by and large that it has the advantages of the Chinese patent medicine for being fairly safe from any fallout but capable of eradicating the illness in the long run, and of the Western medicine for having faster curative effect; hence, believing that the combined preparation offers a better therapy. As described by the interviewees:

"… I am more in favour of combining western medicine with Chinese patent medicine, so that it treats both the symptoms and the root of the problem… " (27, male, master's degree)

"… I don't have inclination, as long as it can cure the disease… " (27, female, bachelor's degree)

"… I would choose Chinese patent medicine when it is a slow case, because it has less side effects… But if it is urgent, I go for western medicine for quick relief… " (25, male, bachelor's degree)

"… both have pros and cons… It is safer to take Chinese patent medicine but less effective… Western medicine works the other way round, but its side effects worry me. (31, female, junior college graduate)

5.3.3.2 Guidance Needed in Shopping for Drugs

A prevailing problem with using Chinese patent medicine is the heavy presence of the Chinese medicine terminology in the instructions concerning functions, indications, etc., which are not easy to grasp for general consumers to ascertain whether some drug suits their cases or not. Some interviewees said:

"… [regarding] Chinese patent medicine… I don't understand the efficacy part, not sure how it works … " (26, male, master's degree)

"… [regarding] Chinese patent medicine… I wish there were detailed explanations to help me understand Chinese medicine theory… " (27, male, bachelor's degree)

"… [regarding] Chinese patent medicine … I need to find out if it agrees with me … " (26, female, bachelor's degree)

Furthermore, Chinese patent medicine, most being of compound preparation, the consumers find their composition too complicated and the instructions overwhelmingly detailed. As interviewees said:

"… [regarding] Chinese patent medicine… I think it has more side effects than western medicine; so the pharmacist should provide clearer guide on how to stave it off …" (48, female, senior high school graduate)

"… [Regarding drug instructions] Chinese patent medicine needs it all the more … because the composition is so complex…" (36, male, bachelor's degree)

Besides, quite a number of OTC Chinese patent medicines share the same generic name but sell in diverse price range with different brands. In recent years, new dose patterns of Chinese patent medicine have increasingly emerged, which has caused such price differences and perplexed the consumers. As described by one interviewee:

> "… [regarding] Chinese patent medicine … many of them look the same but for so different prices … so weird … " (24 male, junior college graduate)

With respect to Western medicine, drug safety is the primary concern of the vast majority of the consumers. There is an urgent need for pharmacists' help with the safety precautions. Some interviewees thought that

> "… [regarding] western medicine … has more adverse effects [than Chinese patent medicine], not sure how to take it safely… " (29 male, Master's degree)

> "… [regarding] western medicine … may cause harm to the body, and nowadays many of them are damaging to the kidneys … " (43 male, junior high school graduate)

> "… [regarding] western medicine … too many side effects. Wondering if it could be made less without reducing its efficacy …" (36 male, bachelor's degree)

On the other hand, those better educated consumers would welcome more information about the drug composition as well as the functions and indications detailed in the instruction, which was described as

> "… [regarding] western medicine … its pharmacological effects are complicated, which I want to know …" (27 male, bachelor's degree)

> "… [regarding] western medicine …its main components, side effects, adverse reactions, etc. are not clear to me" (37 male, bachelor's degree)

> "… [regarding] western medicine … the composition and functions, [not sure] what is what…" (33 female, bachelor's degree)

Based on the responses from the greater majority of all the consumers on our interviews, there seems little discrepancy between the opinions of Chinese patent medicine- and Western medicine goers that guidance of doctors and pharmacists on how to use drugs is necessary. The existing community pharmacies tend to offer a line of OTC drugs in great varieties for curing the same illness, which is also a cause of confusion to the consumers. The interviewees said:

> "… [regarding both Chinese patent medicine and western medicine] advice on drug use is needed … Nowadays there are a wide variety of drugs for curing the same disease to choose from, but one can't tell which is the most helpful for one's case…" (24 female, junior college graduate)

> "… [regarding both Chinese medicine and western medicine] guidance on drug use is needed… explanations on dosage, curative effects, warnings and precautions, are all needed." (45 male, junior college graduate)

5.3.3.3 Medication Instructions

The consumers of Chinese patent medicine have complained about excessive use of special technical terms in drug instructions, which prevent them from getting pertinent information. As mentioned by the interviewees:

> "… [regarding] Chinese patent medicine … what are the properties and effects … the distinction between wind-cold and wind-heat types, can't tell … " (29 male, Master's degree)

> "… directions on using Chinese patent medicine are not quite comprehensible… too many professional terms to see the right remedy for the symptom…" (27 female, bachelor's degree)

> "… [regarding] Chinese patent medicine … Chinese medical terms are hard to understand… " (34 female, junior college graduate)

Some consumers point out instructions for Chinese patent medicine are not quite clear and complete in meaning with frequent instances of vague expressions occurring. As described by an interviewee:

> "… [regarding drug instructions for Chinese patent medicine] … quite a bit are missing or, otherwise confusing …" (42 male, university graduate)

As well, there is also the issue of too many medical terms found in the instructions for Western medicine. As described by an interviewee:

> "… [regarding] western medicine … pharmaceutical particulars are just too elaborate…" (27 male, bachelor's degree)

On the other hand, quite a number of Western drug instructions for the consumers in China are copied from the pharmaceutical manufacturing companies in both content and format. Such marketed non-prescription Western drugs had gone through multiple times of clinical experiments, containing a large amount of the relevant data as a result; yet too complicated and hard for the consumers to grab the needed information straight away. The interviewees said:

> "… [regarding] western medicine … instructions are too long-winded, mostly beyond me." (42, male, bachelor's degree)

> "… [regarding] western medicine [instructions] …not understandable, full of foreign language, content looks just the same, so hard to decide…" (47, male, senior high school graduate)

Without recalculating the afore-mentioned factors of various kinds that interfere with eliciting information from medication directions, it can be concluded that the problem in comprehending instructions does not just pertain to Chinese medicine consumers.

> "… too many technical terms to understand…" (24, male, bachelor's degree)

> "… somewhat incomprehensible … mostly full of medical terms, not totally clear …" (26, female, bachelor's degree)

"… something like interactive effects…[I] don't get it…" (27, male, bachelor's degree)

"… [I] have questions on both [Chinese patent medicine and western medicine instructions] … especially contraindications, warnings, interactions with other drugs … nothing seems quite understandable …" (31, female, junior college graduate)

5.4 Challenges and Suggestions

The case study presented above is attempted to offer a general picture of how qualitative interview method could be applied in Chinese medicine research. At the same time, we hope to have highlighted the need for anticipating some major challenges that confront the researchers in practice.

Challenge of Minimizing Cultural Bias in Sampling Studies in Chinese medicine are intrinsically linked with Chinese culture in one way or another. Respondents' upbringing and schooling have shaped their views, extreme or balanced, of Chinese culture, which consequently affect their attitude, understanding and acceptance of Chinese medicine. As a result, cultural bias is unavoidable in applying qualitative approach in Chinese medicine study. Researchers are obligated to bear this in mind when making decision on sampling.

Challenge of Designing and Asking Interview Questions Related to the challenges of sampling bias, how to design and ask interview questions is another major challenge. It is inevitable that researchers tend to ask questions containing words like '*Yin*', '*Yang*', '*Shanghuo*', '*Tixu*', etc., which are specific terms of Chinese medicine, but sound strange to interviewees who are not familiar with Chinese medicine.

Challenge of Developing Intangible Concepts and Constructs Even if researchers have accomplished their interviews as planned, they may still encounter problems when it comes to the data analysis. To validate a known theory or articulate a new one, researchers need to develop theoretical concepts and constructs from their heavy interview notes and other quantitative materials. But they may find the interview record full of intricacies of Chinese medicine, which can be difficult to understand by people who have no pertinent knowledge. Or they may find the themes developed from interview notes incompatible with the mainstream field that is dominated by Western medicine.

There is no immediate remedy for rising to the challenges; however, from the case study above, some suggestions could be provided for the future development and application of qualitative interviewing for research into Chinese medicine.

Apply a Comparative Research Strategy n most cases, interviewees treat Chinese medicine as a mirror of Western medicine. Therefore, for a qualitative study of Chinese medicine, comparative research approach is deemed appropriate and effective. Researchers can use Western medicine as a point of reference to elicit and comprehend interviewee's notion of Chinese medicine. The design of our project discussed in this chapter serves as a case in point.

Get Your Interview Protocol Well Prepared Owing to the difficulties of clarifying the cultural factors in Chinese medicine, it is crucial to design interview protocol appropriate for Chinese medicine. Researchers need to prepare their interview protocol according to not only literature but empirical data, for example, preliminary exchanges with doctors and patients. In addition, pilot interview is a must for testing the protocol on trial.

Integrate Views of Chinese Medicine with Western Medicine in Data Analysis In the past, researchers in Chinese medicine would define and explore their research objective from the viewpoint of Chinese medicine, which caused the problems of validity and alienation in dialogue with Western medicine. Such problems become more significant in qualitative research. Thus, when applying qualitative interview method to Chinese medicine study, a balanced view of Chinese medicine and Western medicine is critical to a project. By interpreting research objective, results and findings from the perspectives of both Chinese medicine and Western medicine, researchers will gain wider acceptance of their research contributions by members of different cultural and education backgrounds in the field. Moreover, it will help researcher to deepen their thinking to open new avenues of inquiring into patients and their diseases.

5.5 Summary

While qualitative interview has its special strengths in studying Chinese medicine, its practical application is still in its infancy. Looking ahead, we anticipate that researchers will benefit more from using this method to design and implement their research projects that target different subjects and objects (e.g. patients, doctors, pharmacists, nurses, etc.). Applied to studying Chinese medicine not only in the Chinese context but within other sociocultural contexts as well, qualitative interview is expected to become a modus operandi for researchers from different cultural backgrounds in their studies related to Chinese medicine. Only through such extensive experimentation and realization, systematic and practical guidelines will be developed to facilitate qualitative research on Chinese medicine.

Acknowledgments The authors would like to thank University of Macau for its support for this project (MYRG2015-00072-ICMS-QRCM).

References

1. Malterud K. Qualitative research: standards, challenges, and guidelines. Lancet. 2001;358 (9280):483–8.
2. Pope C, Mays N. Qualitative methods in health research. In: Pope C, Mays N, editors. Qualitative research in health care. 3rd ed. Oxford: Blackwell Publishing; 2006. p. 1–11.
3. Giacomini MK, Cook DJ. Group E-BMW. Users' guides to the medical literature: XXIII. Qualitative research in health care A. Are the results of the study valid? JAMA. 2000;284(3): 357–62.
4. Giacomini MK, Cook DJ. Group E-BMW. Users' guides to the medical literature: XXIII. Qualitative research in health care B. What are the results and how do they help me care for my patients? JAMA. 2000;284(4):478–82.
5. Britten N. Qualitative interviews. In: Pope C, Mays N, editors. Qualitative research in health care. 3rd ed. Oxford: Blackwell Publishing; 2006. p. 12–20.
6. Coyne IT. Sampling in qualitative research. Purposeful and theoretical sampling; merging or clear boundaries? J Adv Nurs. 1997;26(3):623–30.
7. Marshall MN. Sampling for qualitative research. Fam Pract. 1996;13(6):522–6.
8. Malterud K, Siersma VD, Guassora AD. Sample size in qualitative interview studies: guided by information power. Qual Health Res. 2015:1049732315617444.
9. Ritchie J, Spencer L. Qualitative data analysis for applied policy research. In: Bryman A, Burgess RG, editors. Analyzing qualitative data. London: Routledge; 2002. p. 305–29.
10. Braun V, Clarke V. Using thematic analysis in psychology. Qual Res Psychol. 2006;3(2): 77–101.
11. Pope C, Ziebland S, Mays N. Analysing qualitative data. BMJ. 2000;320(7227):114–6.
12. Bradley EH, Curry LA, Devers KJ. Qualitative data analysis for health services research: developing taxonomy, themes, and theory. Health Serv Res. 2007;42(4):1758–72.

Chapter 6
A Need for Standard Data Collection Procedure in Studies on Traditional Chinese Medicine

Hutcha Sriplung and Xuesong Yang

Abstract Chinese medicine (CM) practitioners usually base clinical decisions on their own experience and judgment. Although western medicine is now much dependent on objective measurements by medical equipment, in some fields such as in psychology and psychiatry, and in taking clinical information from history and physical examination, subjective measurements are still used. However, the difference is the use of standard data collection procedure. When a CM practitioner bases their collection of clinical information on a theoretical goal, information that fits one's mind set is of concern and that does not fit one's aim is subconsciously screened out. With this practice, the clinical information is biased toward a set of diseases and related *zhengs* in mind. The standardization procedures for clinical data collection can be applied to CM to solve this problem. This chapter will present scientific methods to make standard data collection procedures such as Delphi technique in creating a standard data collection procedure and the tests of its reliability. Objective domain-based technique for questionnaire and checklist design will be discussed. The essential steps in these procedures to ensure objective measurement are the independency of theories and expert opinions and the application of scientific validation methods of the resulting data collection forms. When the results of the studies using the discussed methods confirm the traditional theories, the theoretical foundation of such the disease or *zheng* in CM is confirmed. When studies consistently disagree with the traditional theories, objective modification of theories makes CM moving forward and gets acceptance by western medicine.

Keywords Standard data collection · Delphi technique · Questionnaire · Checklist

H. Sriplung (✉)
Epidemiology Unit, Faculty of Medicine, Prince of Songkla University, Songkhla, Thailand
e-mail: hutcha.s@psu.ac.th

X. Yang
Dermatology Department, Yunnan Provincial Hospital of Traditional Chinese Medicine, Kunming, China
e-mail: imfanjimmy@sohu.com

S. Leung and H. Hu (eds.), *Evidence-based Research Methods for Chinese Medicine*, DOI 10.1007/978-981-10-2290-6_6

6.1 Introduction

For thousands of year, traditional eastern medicine (TEM), mainly used in China (Chinese Medicine, CM), Korea, Mongolia, and Tibet, has founded its theories and practices on subjective clinical information collected by observation of patients' history, living environment, body foundation, clinical signs and symptoms of diseases, pulse palpation, and other clinical evaluation methods. China is the country that has been conducting studies in CM, so the author uses the word CM to cover the ideas and practices in TEM as a whole.

In the far past, western medicine (WM) and medical practices in other countries in Asia, such as Ayurvedic medicine in India, and traditional medicine in Southeast Asia used the same concept of clinical symptoms and signs to classify diseases as well. Diseases were believed to be caused by internal imbalance, response to the environmental change, as well as the supernatural power such as miasma, curse, and intoxication [1]. At that time, CM and Ayurvedic medicine seem to base on a firmer background of disease concept than that of the western medicine.

6.1.1 A Big Leap in Western Medicine

Around early to late nineteenth century during the time of John Snow [1, 2], Louis Pasteur [3], Robert Koch [4], and Joseph Lister [5], the discovery of germs and germ infection as the cause of infectious diseases changed the classification of the disease in western medicine to the cause of diseases rather than the classification based on presenting symptoms and signs of diseases. Such the paradigm shift in disease classification as well as the growth of material science has laid the western style of medicine very solid background for theories of diseases.

While WM practices have moved toward objective measurements, it seems like CM has been far lacking behind. CM practitioners still base their clinical decision on their own experience and judgment.

However, there are still some diseases such as psychotic disease and psychological problems that leave rooms for doctor's judgment for diagnosis and treatment of the diseases or disorders based on patients' symptoms and signs. In these conditions, practitioners take clinical information from history taken by patient interview, physical examination, and use subjective decision in which inconsistency in diagnosis and clinical decision varies by presentation of patients' symptoms and signs and also by doctors' experience.

6.1.2 The Difference Between WM and CM

However, the difference in the practice among CM and psychiatric practitioners is the use of standard data collection procedure. Various screening tests for psychiatric problems have been developed and tested for reliability and validity in systematic ways. Attitude, belief, and anything related to personal judgment fall into this phenomenon as well. Wealth and health statuses are rather subjective measurement. Health professions know this problem and have tried to develop methods to tackle this uncertainty of measurement.

One of the serious pitfalls in CM in clinical data collection is the use of its theory to guide history taking procedure, physical examination, and in collection of all other clinical information from the patients. When one uses a theoretical goal to collect clinical information, information that fits one's mind set is of concern and that does not fit one's aim is screened out. With this convention, the clinical information is biased toward a set of diseases and related *zheng* in mind. Other information that suggest the possibility of another set of diseases being intentionally excluded. The approach of western medicine nowadays is to make use of a check list of all relevant information formulated by various statistical techniques so that the goal is not set as the disease or *zheng* in mind. Such standardization procedures for clinical data collection in western medicine can be applied in as well.

We are presenting scientific methods to make standard data collection procedures such as Delphi technique in creating a standard data collection procedure and the tests of its reliability. Objective-domain-based technique for questionnaire and checklist design will be discussed as well. The essential steps in these procedures to ensure objective measurement are the independency of theories and expert opinions and the application of scientific validation methods of the resulting data collection forms.

6.2 Standardization of Data Collection

Standardized data collection tool is an agreed instrument which enables data concerning patients, therapists, and/or healthcare settings and approaches to be collected unambiguously by a range of practitioners in a number of different clinical settings of clinical practice of services collecting and recording [6]. The standardization is the process to ensure that the data collected are reliable, precise, and reproducible. It is true that standardization of data collection cannot avoid uncertainty of the data by subjective decision. However, there are processes in minimizing uncertainty of measurement using the standard data collection methods.

In WM, standardized data collection tools may be in descriptive document where essential items are written in the medical records, data collection forms, or electronic devices. The format of data collection tools does not matter when all the essential information is collected. The important issue is how the essential information is summarized and who decide that the information is important and complete.

In CM, practitioners usually note the patient data on the medical records. CM practitioners base their decision on what to note and how to get the information on the theory of CM they are using. The problem in this practice is that there are different theories used in different text books or schools they graduated from, and the different in experiences of the CM practitioners themselves.

6.2.1 Delphi Technique

The Delphi technique is named after the Pythia prophecy, also known as the Oracle of Delphi, in the Temple of Apollo at Delphi, a place located on the slopes of Mount Parnassus in the ancient Greece. Many famous Greek leaders came to have their questions answered at Delphi.

The Delphi technique used nowadays is not the mythical one mentioned above. It mainly developed by Dalkey and Helmer at the Rand Corporation in the 1950s [7, 8], which is a widely used method for achieving convergence of opinion concerning real-world knowledge solicited from experts within certain topic areas. The Delphi technique is designed as a group communication process that aims at conducting detailed illumination and discussions of a specific issue in various fields. The technique attempts to address the question of what should be expected in case a situation occurs [9].

The Delphi technique is well suited as a means and method for building a convergent agreement using a series of questionnaire to collect data from a panel of selected informants. The process requires multiple iterations designed to develop a convergence of opinion concerning a specific topic. Theoretically, the Delphi process can be iterated until consensus is determined to have been achieved or none of the experts changes the idea. However, studies suggested that three iterations are often sufficient to collect the important information and to reach a convergence in most cases even in different topics of study [8, 10, 11].

There is a series of steps to construct a checklist that can be applied to the standard data collection form development. We suggest an approach consisted of five predefined steps [10, 12–15].

(1) *Literature review*: A thorough literature review must be done so that a list of symptoms and signs related to the disease under study is formulated. There are different textbooks and schools of CM, those written or taught in those textbooks and schools must not be omitted.
(2) *Checklist design*: The researchers/developers draft the initial checklist in which symptoms and signs should be systematically grouped in domains for ease of making decision by experts.
(3) *Scores of the items*: Experts are asked to score their opinions on the items in semi-quantitative scales (see the next topic). The semi-quantitative opinions can be one of the 3, 5, or 10 Likert-type scales, or they can be in a visual analog scale.

(4) *Expert consensus*: Now that the initial checklist is made, send the checklist to a group of no less than five experts to review and score it in at least three rounds. The developers must ask their opinions if any missing items should be added. Experts must be distributed in different schools of CM. The details of Delphi process are discussed later.
(5) *Finalization*: After finishing Delphi process, the results must be published, disseminated, implemented, and updated at interval.

The Delphi process is a series of activities to accomplish the conclusion of the idea or a checklist of symptoms and signs of the disease of interest in CM. In drafting a checklist, one may review the literatures and textbooks and design a checklist by oneself. The problem of the action is the acceptance by experts and practitioners. Being an expert is not the exception. To avoid this problem, it is necessary to have experts and practitioners to get involved in the process. The Delphi process to ensure valid results includes the following steps.

(1) *Setting up a steering committee*: The researchers must set up a steering committee to control the quality of whole development process and determine the contents of the checklist. The committee members must be senior researchers who have authority in CM field. It is not necessary that they are in the field of study and must not be the member of informant experts.
(2) *Tasks of steering committee*: Their tasks are to give the direction, to help in any steps that the researchers request, and to make sure that the researchers are not misconducting. The steering committee must discuss with the researchers to approve the final list of experts and also approve the results of literature search, the initial checklist, and facilitate the contact of expert panel through their authority.
(3) *Roles of expert panel*: The expert panel must clearly know the aims of the study and agree to complete all rounds of the discussion. They must know that they themselves are also the subjects of the study.
(4) *Rounds of Delphi process*: In traditional Delphi process, it is advised that the process should begin with open-ended questions [16]. In this chapter where we are going to make a structural checklist, it is necessary to start with a structured initial one. The researchers are responsible to draft an initial checklist and distribute to experts who are approved by the steering committee. The researchers are also collect their opinions and summarize the results of the first round and send the feedback to them and ask for the second round of their opinions. In summarization of the results of the first round, researchers must set the threshold of the response before hand. Any items that get an average score below the threshold would be cut from the second round of the checklist. Such process and threshold must be known by the expert panel at the invitation to join the study. Repeat the process in the third round. As mentioned earlier that three iterations are usually enough to get a high intra-rater agreement even the inter-rater agreement is not high [10], the results of the second and third rounds are usually similar and the fourth round is not necessary.

(5) *Summary reports*: Researchers must report back the results of the study to all members of the expert panel and the steering committee. Together with the report, a letter of thanks arid appreciation of their help should be sent.

For clinical use, it is easier to use when the checklist consists of items with answers yes or no, present or absent. However, there are some cases that the answers should be graded where the knowledge of constructing a semi-quantitative answer described below is required. Thus, the final checklist for clinical use is not the one that the expert panels see but is a practical checklist that is easy to use by practitioners.

In summary, the Delphi technique is time and effort consuming procedure. However, it is necessary if one needs a checklist of symptoms and signs in CM that is accepted by the majority of the CM practitioner, irrespective of textbooks they are using or the school from which they were graduated.

6.3 Construction of a Semi-quantitative Measurement

Some variables are in nominal scale and mutually exclusive. In this case, a semi-quantitative measurement is not appropriate. For example, a patient can be male or female but not in between the two. For allergy, a series of questions to explore which allergen the patient exposed in the last few days, such as whether the patient recently ate seafood, can be answered as yes or no. The amount of exposure is not important in finding the potential allergen. In this situation, a binomial measurement is suitable.

However, there are a lot more clinical symptoms and signs that the extent of the phenomenon, i.e., the exposure to external environment and the manifestation of a disease, can be graded with a quantitative measurement obtained from a medical equipment such as body temperature and blood sugar level. However, there are a number of gradable clinical manifestations that need interpretation by doctor's observation. In this case, a semi-quantitative measurement is needed.

A semi-quantitative measurement is the procedure to transform qualitative measurement in detecting the presence or absence of a subjective observation to provide a numeric representation of the amount of the observed phenomenon. A binomial measurement of the presence or absence of a phenomenon of interest is graded into a range of score for the observed event. The benefit of this method is to make room for observers to state an uncertainty they observe between the presence and absence of the occurrence of that symptom or sign. In fact, in many cases observers are sure that the event is absent or present. In situation that they are not certain to state the extremes, they have an opportunity to say that the fact is likely to be somewhere between the two ends.

On the other hand, the semi-quantitative assessment is also used in interpretation of the results in scientific measurement in percentage or continuous scales that are hard to interpret into a few categories, i.e., low, medium, and high. In this case, uncertainty occurs around the cutpoints as well. This phenomenon is not important to CM since it also occurs in results from medical equipment and statistical analysis in WM.

Even one cannot avoid uncertainty of the semi-quantitative measurement, it is better to state the intermediate or indeterminate decision rather than to force the evidence to be on an extreme side of binomial determination. Some may prefer Likert-type scales of 1 to 3, 5, 10, or 100 in measuring different phenomena. Some may use a visual analog scale (VAS) where observers of patients can mark their decision on the symptom or sign on a straight line where 0 and 10 or 100 are on the two opposite ends. In measurement of severity of pain, doctors in WM usually use a VAS score and 0 means no pain at all and 10 or 100 means the severity of pain that the patient cannot tolerate.

The use of semi-quantitative measurement is clear when a doctor wants to follow a clinical presentation in a long period of time. It is easy to follow the change in ordinal or continuous scales than in a binomial scale. CM practitioners can adopt such a concept to evaluate the presence of a phenomenon to an ordinal or continuous scale of its severity and use the score in statistical analysis.

CM practitioners may feel uncomfortable to classify *zheng* as a probability with uncertainty as shown above. However, in clinical practice of CM, one can see variability of signs, symptoms, and *zheng* in a patient. With this method, it is easy in describing the change in these things over time. And it also allows CM practitioners to communicate the *zheng* diagnosis in the way that a patient has got moderate degree of this *zheng* and some degree of another or others at the same time.

6.4 Statistical Methods for Grouping of Signs and Symptoms

The presence of a group of signs and symptoms of patients, and probably with history of past exposure to climate or diet, leads to *zheng* classification of a disease and diagnosis of a disease. It is possible that the classification of *zhengs* and diseases is different from one to another school of CM, and it may change when systematic analysis of signs and symptoms is evaluated by systematic methods using statistics of grouping.

There are a series of statistical methods to solve grouping problems of clinical manifestations of a disease to identify underlying *zheng* classification. Usually, we use statistical models in the group of latent class analysis and cluster analysis. Other appropriate models can be applied whenever they can group sets of variable with reasonable statistical presumptions and constrains.

6.4.1 Latent Class Analysis

Latent class analysis (LCA) is a statistical method for identifying unmeasured class membership among subjects in a dataset using categorical and/or continuous observed variables. LCA procedure defines latent classes by the criterion of 'conditional independence.' This means that each variable is statistically independent of every other variable within each latent class. For example, within a latent class corresponding to a distinct syndrome, the presence/absence of one symptom is viewed as unrelated to presence/absence of all others. Alternative models were described by Lindsay et al. [17].

The study of Yang et al. [18] was an example of the use of LCA on dichotomous outcomes. *Zheng* classification of psoriasis was evaluated using this method on a standardized clinical checklist developed by the Delphi technique [10]. Three *zhengs* were identified and the difference from those documented in the textbooks was discussed. In Yang's study, dichotomous nature of signs and symptoms was used. For grade characteristics such as tongue coating, they transformed the grades into a series of binomial variables, i.e., thing and thick tongue coating to the presence of thin tongue coating—yes or no, thick tongue coating—yes or no.

Further derivation of LCA is the latent tree model (LTM) described in detail by Zhang et al. [19, 20]. In-depth explanation of the statistical methods of both LCA and LTM is skipped since the aim of this chapter is on standardization of data collection not on statistical analysis.

6.4.2 Cluster Analysis

Cluster analysis is a multivariate method which aims to classify a sample of subjects (or objects) on the basis of a set of measured variables into a number of groups in which similar subjects are placed [21]. It is used in various fields in sciences. An example where the method is used in the field of psychiatry is to characterize patients on the basis of clusters of symptoms. In public health, it is used to identify disease outbreaks. It can also be applied to identify clusters of signs and symptoms which relate to *zhengs* in a disease [22]. Cluster analysis is also used in classification of Chinese herbs and network of herbs used in some diseases [23, 24].

References

1. Tognotti E. The dawn of medical microbiology: germ hunters and the discovery of the cause of cholera. J Med Microbial. 2011:60(Pt 4):555–8. doi:10.1099/jmn.0.025700-0.
2. Lippi D, Gotuzzo E. The greatest steps towards the discovery of Vibrio cholerae. Clin Microbiol Infect. 2014;20(3):191–5. doi:10.1111/1469-0691.12390.
3. Toledo-Pereyra LH. Louis Pasteur surgical revolution. J Invest Slug. 2009;22(2):82–7. doi:10.1080/08941930902794729.

4. Blevins SM, Bronze MS. Robert Koch and the 'golden age' of bacteriology. Int J Infect Dis. 2010;14(9):e744–51. doi:10.1016/j.ijid.2009.12.003.
5. Toledo-Pereyra LH. Joseph Lister's surgical revolution. J Invest Surg. 2010;23(5):241–3. doi:10.3109/08941939.2010.520574.
6. Moore AP, Bryant EC, Olivier GWJ. Development and use of standardised data collection tools to support and inform musculoskeletal practice. Man Ther. 2012;17(6):489–96. doi:10.1016/j.math.2012.07.008.
7. Dalkey NC, Helmer O. An experimental application of the Delphi method to the use of experts. Manag Sci. 1963;9(3):458–67.
8. Hsu C-C, Sandford BA. The Delphi technique: making sense of consensus. Pract Assess Res Eval. 2007;12(10):1–7.
9. Miller LE. Determining what could/should be: The Delphi technique and its application. Paper presented at the meeting of the 2006 annual meeting of the Mid-Western Educational Research Association, Columbus, Ohio. 2006.
10. Yang X, Chongsuvivatwong V. McNeil E, Ye J, Ouyang X, Yang E, Srip lung H. Developing a diagnostic checklist of traditional Chinese medicine symptoms and signs for psoriasis: a Delphi study. Chin Med. 2013;8(1):10. doi:10.1186/1749-8546-8-10.
11. Witt CM, Aickin M, Cherkin D, Che CT, Elder C, Flower A, et al. Effectiveness guidance document (EGD) for Chinese medicine trials: a consensus document. Trials. 2014;15:169. doi:10.1186/1745-6215-15-169.
12. Schmutz J, Eppich WJ, Hoffmann F, Heimberg E, Manser T. Five steps to develop checklists for evaluating clinical performance: an integrative approach. Acad Med. 2014;89(7):996–1005. doi:10.1097/ACM.0000000000000289.
13. Mullen PM. Delphi: myths and reality. J Health Organ Manag. 2003;17(1):37–52.
14. Pietersma S, de Vries M, van den Akker-van Made ME. Domains of quality of life: results of a three-stage Delphi consensus procedure among patients, family of patients, clinicians, scientists and the general public. Qual Life Res. 2014;23(5):1543–56. doi:10.1007/s11136-013-0578-3.
15. Shi N, Zhong LL, Han X, Ziea IC, Ng B, Bian Z, Lu A. Enhanced evidence-based Chinese medicine clinical practice guidelines in Hong Kong: a study protocol for three common diseases. Evid Based Complement Altern Med. 2015;2015:482706. doi:10.1155/2015/482706.
16. Custer RL, Scarcella JA, Stewart BR. The modified Delphi technique: a rotational modification. J Vocat Tee Educ. 1999;15(2):1–10.
17. Lindsay B, Clogs CC, Grego J. Semiparametric estimation in the Rasch model and related exponential response models, including a simple latent class model for item analysis. J Am Stat Assoc. 1991;86(413):96–107.
18. Yang X, Chongsuvivatwong V. Lerkiatbundit S, Ye J, Ouyang X, Yang E, Sriplung H. Identifying the Zheng in psoriatic patients based on latent class analysis of raditional Chinese medicine symptoms and signs. Chin Med. 2014;9(1):1. doi:10.1186/1749-8546-9-1.
19. Zhang NL, Yuan S, Chen T, Wang Y. Latent tree models and diagnosis in traditional Chinese medicine. Artif Intell Med. 2008;42(3):229–45.
20. Zhang NL, Yuan S, Chen T, Wang Y. Statistical validation of traditional chinese medicine theories. J Ahem Complement Med. 2008;14(5):583–7. doi:10.1089/acm.2007.7019.
21. Everitt BS. Cluster analysis. Chichester, West Sussex, U.K.: Wiley; 2011.
22. Tao F, Lu H, Oppert JM, Basdevant A. MENG may contribute to obesity phenotypes based on body composition: a pilot study on the traditional Chinese medicine approach. Evid Based Complement Altemat Med. 2014;2014:580803. doi:10.1155/2014/580803.
23. Pang J, Yang M, Fu J, Zhao X, van Wijk E, Wang M, Liu Y, Zhou X, Fan H, Han J. Classification of Chinese herbs based on the cluster analysis of delayed luminescence. Luminescence. 2015. doi:10.1155/2014/580803.
24. Chen HY, Lin YH, Hu S, Yang SH, Chen JL, Chen YC. Identifying Chinese herbal medicine network for eczema: implications from a nationwide prescription database. Evid Based Complement Altemat Med. 2015;2015:347164. doi:10.1155/2015/347164.

Chapter 7
Methods for Assessment of Interrater Reliability for Diagnosis and Intervention in Traditional Chinese Medicine Studies

Arthur Sá Ferreira and Ingrid Jardim Azeredo Souza Oliveira

Abstract Traditional medicines experienced an increasing interest in theoretical, experimental, and clinical research since its recognition in the Alma-Ata Declaration. Particularly, Chinese medicine (CM) was developed by a society geographic, social, and culturally different from the Western community during the last 3000 years. The diagnostic process of CM has a unique feature: patterns, the counterpart of Western diseases, are identified through a process named *pattern differentiation*. The collection of clinical manifestations of an individual is obtained using four examinations known as inspection, auscultation-olfaction, inquiry, and palpation. As a corollary, CM diagnosis is considered as subjective because only the five senses are used to gather meaningful clinical data and must be interpreted by an expert; no equipment or diagnostic exam was developed for collecting data for pattern differentiation until the last decades. Pattern differentiation comprises a procedure subjected to errors as any other diagnostic system, but this variability in diagnosis might have consequences: different patterns might lead to distinct treatment choices such as herbs or acupoints selection. In contrast with Western medicine that has treatment protocols for various diseases, there are no defined protocols of acupoints for patterns because of the personalized aspect of CM's diagnostic process and the possibility of selecting acupoints using a variety of criteria. Therefore, it is important to assess simultaneously the amount of agreement—mainly among different raters—for CM diagnosis and the diagnostic accuracy for pattern differentiation to determine the validity of this traditional system in both clinical and research scenarios. In this sense, high interrater agreement (i.e. the degree to which raters achieve identical results when performing the same assessment under similar conditions) and diagnostic accuracy (i.e. the rate of correct diagnosis) are important characteristics of any model used for health classification. Previous studies investigated the agreement for pattern differentiation and/or for acupuncture prescription,

A.S. Ferreira (✉) · I.J.A.S. Oliveira
Laboratory of Computational Simulation and Modeling in Rehabilitation, Augusto Motta University Center, Rio de Janeiro, RJ, Brazil
e-mail: arthurde@unisuamdoc.com.br

I.J.A.S. Oliveira
e-mail: guigarden@yahoo.com.br

S. Leung and H. Hu (eds.), *Evidence-based Research Methods for Chinese Medicine*, DOI 10.1007/978-981-10-2290-6_7

though they present important limitations either from the traditional or scientific perspective. A lack of calculating and reporting statistical measures of agreement or a lack of investigating the relationship between diagnosis and therapeutic prescription was observed. Finally, the above-cited studies used real human patients, in which the *true pattern* was unknown and therefore it is not possible to assess the diagnostic accuracy with a gold-standard model. This chapter introduces advanced methods for assessing interrater reliability for diagnosis and intervention in CM. More specifically, this chapter discusses the choices of study design and statistical methods for measuring interrater reliability and diagnostic accuracy in the context of pattern differentiation and acupuncture prescription. Sample size calculation and proper agreement coefficients for the multinomial, univariate or multivariate scenarios are presented. The role of computational simulation as a gold-standard method is also addressed. Finally, computational methods for statistical analysis of reliability and diagnostic performance are presented and discussed in the context of reliability and diagnostic accuracy analysis in CM.

Keywords Reliability · Diagnostic performance · Chinese medicine · Rehabilitation

7.1 Introduction

This chapter presents a collection of methods for a study protocol aiming to investigate interrater agreement for pattern differentiation and diagnostic acupoints prescription, as well as diagnostic accuracy for pattern differentiation. In particular, this chapter is designed to help researchers develop study protocols aiming (i) to determine interrater agreement of Chinese medicine (CM) experts for pattern differentiation, (ii) to determine interrater agreement of CM experts for acupoints prescription, and (iii) to determine diagnostic performance of a sample of CM experts. Although this text is not a complete guide to such a task, it is our expectation that the researcher may start designing his/her own study protocol using the recommendations provided herein.

7.2 On the Need for Assessing Reliability and Accuracy

Traditional medicines experienced an increasingly interest in theoretical, experimental, and clinical research since its recognition in the Alma-Ata Declaration [1]. Particularly, Chinese medicine (CM) was developed by a society geographic, social, and culturally different from the Western community during the last 3000 years [2, 3].

The diagnostic process of CM has a unique feature: patterns, the CM's counterpart of Western diseases, are identified through a process named pattern differentiation. The collection of clinical manifestations of an individual—the so-called *manifestation profile*—is obtained using the four examinations, namely inspection, auscultation-olfaction, inquiry, and palpation [4]. As a corollary, the diagnosis is considered as highly subjective because only the five senses are used to gather meaningful clinical data that must be yet interpreted by a CM expert. Interestingly, despite the high advances of early Chinese societies [2], no equipment or diagnostic exam was developed for collecting data for pattern differentiation until Western science meet the Chinese one in the last decades. Though CM practitioners follow systematic–philosophic relationships between the humans and Nature to identify the diagnosis [5], CM's pattern differentiation comprises a procedure subjected to errors as any other diagnostic system.

In Western medical practice, errors are difficult to recognize but are not rare [6–8]. Misdiagnosis, late diagnosis, and no diagnosis are among the types of diagnostic errors most commonly practiced in medicine. Many cases of diagnostic errors are due to difficulties in differentiating between two closely related or similar diagnoses. Nonetheless, they might have very different prognosis or therapeutic options. Likewise, different CM patterns might lead to distinct treatment choices such as herbs combinations and selection of acupoints. In contrast with Western medicine that has treatment protocols for various diseases, there are no defined protocols of acupoints for patterns because of the personalized aspect of CM's diagnostic process and the possibility of selecting acupoints using a variety of criteria [4]. For instance, CM experts are expected to combine several *yin-yang* rules for balancing—or even unbalancing—an acupuncture prescription, including left-right, upper-lower, front-back body parts, generic-specific, and local-distal rules [4].

Therefore, it is important to assess both the amount of agreement for CM diagnosis and the diagnostic accuracy itself to determine the validity of CM intervention in either clinical and research scenarios. In this sense, high agreement—mainly among different raters, i.e., the degree to which raters achieve identical results when performing the same assessment under similar conditions—and diagnostic accuracy are important characteristics of any model used for classification from which health-related decisions are taken.

7.3 What Have We Learned from Previous Research?

Investigation of reliability and diagnostic accuracy are well-established research methods within Western researchers. Nonetheless, experts on CM only drove their attention to this matter very recently. Previous studies investigated the agreement for pattern differentiation and/or for acupuncture prescription [9–17], though they present important limitations either from the CM or scientific perspective. Among these limitations, we might highlight a lack of: calculating and reporting statistical measures of agreement [10–12, 14]; investigating the relationship between diagnosis and therapeutic prescription [11, 13–17]; assessing the influence of diagnostic errors on both agreements of CM experts for pattern differentiation and for acupuncture prescription. Most importantly, the above-mentioned studies used real human patients whom the *true* pattern was unknown beforehand—only the diagnosis of CM expert, which is prone to rater's subjectivity and thus diagnostic error—and thus it is not possible to assess diagnostic accuracy with a *true* gold-standard model.

At this point one, may argue what could be used instead; another starting point is: *simulated* human patients. Simulation of human patients has becoming a very useful practice in several medical fields, with aims varying from education through training to evaluation. As a matter of fact, automated systems have been developed to study the pattern differentiation process, most of them focused in the diagnosis itself and not in the simulation of human patients [18]. To overcome major limitations due to limited availability and fragmented implementations of computational models, a large project on computerization of CM research and practice is ongoing—the SuiteTCM [19]—and some tools are already available from this initiative.

SimTCM[1] is the first simulation tool designed to simulate human patients according to CM patterns using computational models [20]. *SimTCM* is the second generation of simulation models that evolved from the early algorithm for simulation of manifestation profiles (MPSA) [21], which was proposed for simulation of manifestation profiles with known diagnosis, either cases or controls subjects with respect to prevalences of patterns and manifestations. Another interesting computational tool is the pattern differentiation algorithm (PDA), introduced in that same study [21] used an objective criterion for selection of candidate patterns and ranking them as diagnostic hypothesis, namely *explained information*, $F_{\%}$. Simply stating, $F_{\%}$ captures the proportion of manifestations reported by a patient that explains each pattern belonging to a dataset of possible patterns, in the sense that the larger $F_{\%}$ is for a given pattern the higher the possibility that all manifestations reported by the patient belongs to that pattern. In a sequential study [22], PDA incorporated another objective criterion, namely *available information* $N_{\%}$, also used for candidate pattern selection and diagnostic hypotheses ranking. Using the same dataset of 69 *zangfu* patterns in both studies, a statistically significant increase in diagnostic accuracy was found using both PDA's criteria $F_{\%}$ and $N_{\%}$ as compared to $F_{\%}$ alone (accuracy: 94.7 vs. 93.2 %; sensitivity = 89.8 vs. 86.5 %; specificity = 99.5 vs. 99.9 %, respectively; $p < 0.001$). As related to the second criterion, a specific proportion of available information ($N_{\%} = 28.5$ %) was required to achieve the optimal diagnostic accuracy—neither too few nor too many manifestations make easier to diagnosis—which was recommended as a cutoff value.

PDA and MPSA were used to investigate diagnostic errors in pattern differentiation; it was possible only because the true target-pattern of the human patients were *known* a priori from the simulation procedure [23]. In that study, diagnostic outcomes were separated into correct diagnosis, misdiagnosis, or no diagnosis. Testing the pattern differentiation among 73 *zangfu* patterns and using the four examinations the lowest misdiagnosis and no diagnosis rates were observed

[1]Available at http://www.unisuam.edu.br/index.php/downloads-cr.

(6.0 and 1.4 %, respectively) and shared manifestations among dual patterns was identified as an important source of error in pattern differentiation.

Statistical softwares might also be of some help not only for study designing but also evaluating the study's results. An interesting tool is The R Project for Statistical Computing[2] [24], a free software environment that performs statistical computing and generates graphics for visual representation of data. What makes this software interesting—besides being freely available—is that researchers share packages they developed, which are solid grounded in literature. As for reliability and diagnostic accuracy studies, some of the most appealing packages comprise 'blockrand' [25], 'boot' [26], 'caret' [27], 'irr' [28], 'kappaSize' [29], 'psy' [30], and 'xlsx' [31] packages.

7.4 Designing Reliability and Diagnostic Accuracy Studies

Research guidelines have been proposed for a variety of study designs, including reliability and diagnostic accuracy.[3] On the one hand, for assessment of reliability, researchers are strongly recommended to follow the Guidelines for Reporting Reliability and Agreement Studies (GRRAS) [32]. Also, whether the reliability for intervention selection is to be assessed the Standards for Reporting Interventions in Clinical Trials of Acupuncture (STRICTA) [33, 34] is also required, mainly for determining the characteristics of the CM experts enrolled in the study. On the other hand, for assessment of diagnostic accuracy, researchers should follow the Standards for Reporting of Diagnostic Accuracy (STARD) [35]. A general flowchart for reliability studies is presented in Fig. 7.1 and is depicted in the next sections.

7.4.1 Ethical Issues

The first issue to consider for planning studies enrolling human subjects is ethics in research. Any study protocol must be elaborated in accordance with major ethical policies such as the Declaration of Helsinki and national resolutions regarding ethics in research involving humans. Also, the study protocol must receive an approval by the institutional ethics Committee prior to its execution, and reporting the register number of this approval is strongly advised. Another major requirement is that all participants—raters in this case—must be unambiguously informed about the study aims, potential risks, and benefits associated with their participation.

[2]Available at http://www.r-project.org.

[3]Enhancing the QUAlity and Transparency Of health Research (EQUATOR network) available at http://www.equator-network.org.

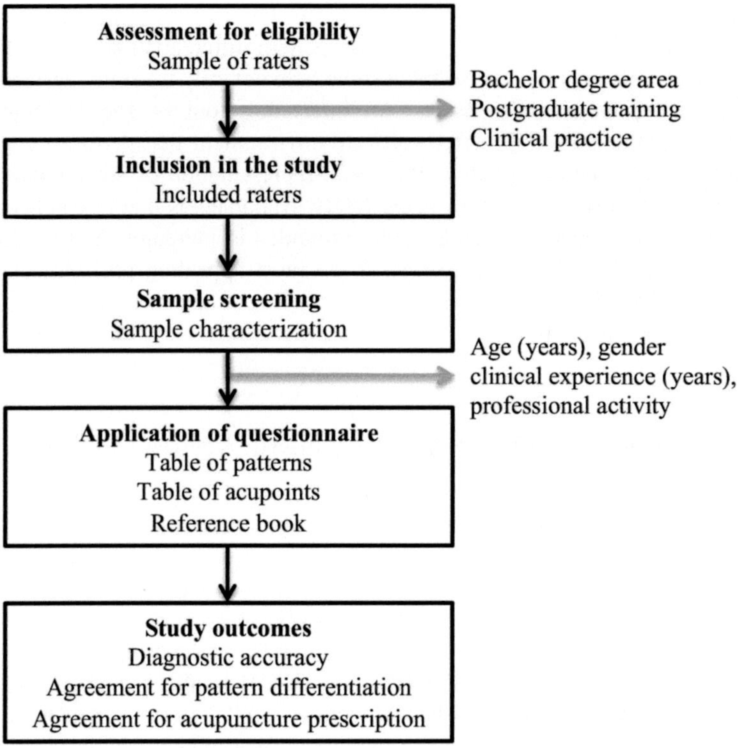

Fig. 7.1 Framework for a study protocol aiming to assess interrater reliability

The signature of an informed consent form agreeing to participate in this study after such explanations certifies this criterion and is mandatory for each rater included in the study.

All above-cited guidelines—GRAAS, STARD, and STRICTA—strongly recommend to collect and provide summary information regarding the sample of raters. More specifically, the duration of training period, and the duration of clinical experience in CM are possible confounders of interrater reliability and diagnostic accuracy.

7.4.2 Sample Size Requirements

Sample size calculations are often disregarded in CM research and the reasons behind this fact are easily speculated: information for calculating sample sizes is not often available in previous studies, and when available the difficulty lies in finding the sample size formula that better suits the plan for statistical analysis as well as the study hypothesis. An additional limitation is that only few computation implementations of formulas for calculating sample sizes are available, making it difficult to the less experienced researcher to correctly estimate the required sample size. Nonetheless, sample size calculations are formal requirements for all guidelines consulted herein.

Let us just not miss the point: sample size calculations are the better way to observe the desired effect size (i.e., difference, correlation, reliability, and accuracy) considering a given type-I (the so-called *significance level* or α, usually established on 5 % or lower) and type-II (the so-called *power of study* or 1-β, usually established on 75 % or higher) errors while avoid spending more resources (i.e. human, time, and financial) than necessary. It must be emphasized that as for reliability and diagnostic accuracy studies, there are *two sample sizes* to be calculated: the sample size of raters *and* the sample size of patients to be diagnosed.

Another important issue to consider is missing data and dropouts. To avoid reducing the study's power due to either one of these reasons, researchers are advised to inflate their minimal sample sizes by a factor of say 10 % or higher depending on the expected rates of respondent raters.

7.5 Sample Size of Raters

The major factor that influences the power of statistical analysis in reliability studies is the number of cases being analyzed by each rater. It is not advantageous to increase too much, the number of raters because the effects on the statistical power and amplitude of confidence intervals are small. It was demonstrated that the number of raters is inversely proportional to the required number of cases, although the saving in sample size rapidly decreases after five raters [36]. Although interrater reliability might be evaluated for two raters only, a minimum sample size of five raters is easily obtained and strongly advised.

It is worth noting that estimates of sample sizes for raters are related to each group being analyzed in the research. This means that if a study protocol aims to compare the reliability between two groups of raters defined by a given factor—say, <5 and ≥ 5 years of clinical practice—each group must present the minimal sample size of raters as estimated.

7.6 Sample Size of Patients

Available formulas implemented in computational models for determining the sample size of cases consider the number of raters, the expected value of agreement against a given null hypothesis (or alternatively, a confidence interval of 95 % [$CI_{95\%}$]), and the number of categories in the studied variable—in this case, the number of possible CM patterns that could be considered as the diagnosis.

It is not clinically relevant to test the null hypothesis H_0: $\kappa_0 = 0.00$ versus $\kappa_0 = \kappa$ because reliability equal to 0 only means that agreement was achieved by chance alone. Therefore, it is strongly recommended to establish a minimal reliability value as the null hypothesis to calculate the sample size and consequently to accept the results as clinically relevant. As a matter of fact, $\kappa = 0.75$ or higher is usually regarded as the lowest yet relevant reliability. Therefore, it is suggested to establish the null hypothesis as $\kappa_0 = 0.75$ with $CI_{95\%} = [0.71; 0.80]$. Yet, because agreement is acknowledged as varying from poor to excellent in CM, a less conservative approach would be to consider the null hypothesis as $\kappa_0 = 0.70$ with $CI_{95\%} = [0.41; 0.99]$.

Sample sizes can be obtained using the R package 'kappaSize' [29] with a basic starting code such as the code in the box below:

```
# Install the required package for sample size
calculation
require("kappaSize")
# Load the package
library(kappaSize)
# Display the reference of the package
print(citation(package = "kappaSize", lib.loc = NULL))
```

Example 1 Consider that a study aims to assess the interrater reliability ($k = 2$) for detecting the presence of a given CM pattern (0 = absentee; 1 = present). Significance level was set at $\alpha = 5$ % and the prevalence at 50 %. Using the confidence interval approach, one may calculate the required sample size to test the null hypothesis $\kappa_0 = 0.70$ with $CI_{95\%} = [0.41; 0.99]$ using the code in the box below:

```
# Display the estimated sample size
print("Confidence interval approach")
print(CIBinary(kappa0=0.70, kappaL=0.41, kappaU=0.99,
props=0.5, raters=2, alpha=0.05))
```

which outputs:

```
[1] "Confidence interval approach"
[2] A minimum of 39 subjects are required for this study
of interobserver agreement
```

Example 2 Consider that another study aims to assess the interrater reliability ($k = 2$) for detecting the presence of a given CM pattern (0 = absentee;

1 = present). Significance level was set at $\alpha = 5\ \%$, the power of the study was set to $\beta = 80\ \%$, and the prevalence at 50 %. Using the power-based approach, one may calculate the required sample size to test the null hypothesis $\kappa_0 = 0.41$ versus $\kappa_1 = 0.70$ replacing those last lines of that code by these in the box below:

```
# Display the estimated sample size
print("Power-based approach")
print(PowerBinary(kappa0=0.75, kappa1=0.41, props=0.55,
raters=2, alpha=0.05, power=0.80))
```

which outputs:

```
[1] "Power-based approach"
[2] A minimum of 30 subjects are required for this study
of interobserver agreement
```

7.6.1 Participants Screening and Admission

The studied sample should be selected from the population of raters, with probabilistic or no probabilistic sampling schemes; the researcher must clearly state the selection method in details no matter the choice made. With the list of raters available, the principal investigator must contact each rater in an independent manner for clarification of the study aims, methods, and presentation of a critical analysis of potential risks and benefits. Raters must be made blinded regarding the results of the other raters enrolled in the same study and to the diagnostic outcomes of the cases to be presented in the questionnaire.

A self-administered questionnaire for sample characterization as well as for checking the adherence for inclusion criteria must be developed prior to data collection. According to the reporting guidelines [33, 34], at least the following questions about personal and professional characteristics of the rater are necessary: age (years), sex, area of graduate course, professional occupation, period of completion of the course of expertise (in years), time (in hours), and duration (in hours) of acupuncture training in the specialization course. Questionnaires must be filled in loco immediately after the participant's admission. Summary data analysis may be conducted only after data collection from all raters.

7.6.2 Eligibility: Inclusion and Exclusion Criteria

General recommendations for inclusion criteria are as follows: (a) bachelor degree (or equivalent) in any health-related course recognized by the National Ministry of Education, including but not limited to medicine, nursing, physical therapy, speech therapy, physician, nutrition, dentistry, psychology, and occupational therapy; (b) graduate or postgraduate training in acupuncture registered at the respective national professional council; (c) clinical practice for at least 1 year; and (d) signature of the informed consent form after reading about the objectives, potential risks and benefits for participating in this research. Other criteria may be added to meet any specific requirements for attaining the study aims.

It is strongly advised that only certified professionals should be enrolled in such studies as raters. The inclusion of raters not yet certified will be only acceptable in case reliability and diagnostic accuracy are studied in the context of education.

It is part of the ethics in research that raters should be excluded from the study upon request to the principal investigator. However, problems might occur in the process of gathering data, which is usually made using questionnaires. Indeed, returning rates of questionnaires may be very low and the number of incomplete questionnaires may be conversely high [37]. Therefore, the most general recommendation is to exclude from the study raters that do not provide answers to all questionnaires.

7.7 Implementing Reliability and Diagnostic Accuracy Studies

At least three steps may be organized for implementing reliability and diagnostic accuracy studies using the framework of simulation. Those steps are depicted in Fig. 7.2 and are explained in details in subsequent sections.

7.7.1 Obtaining a Valid Domain of Patterns for Diagnosis

There are at least two requirements to work with simulation of patients. The first one is a database with the patterns of interest for research. Current research advocates the paradigm 'pattern|disease' [38], which is based on the concept that a given disease (in the Western sense) may present a limited set of CM patterns. Therefore, the database of patterns must contain all possible patterns that were

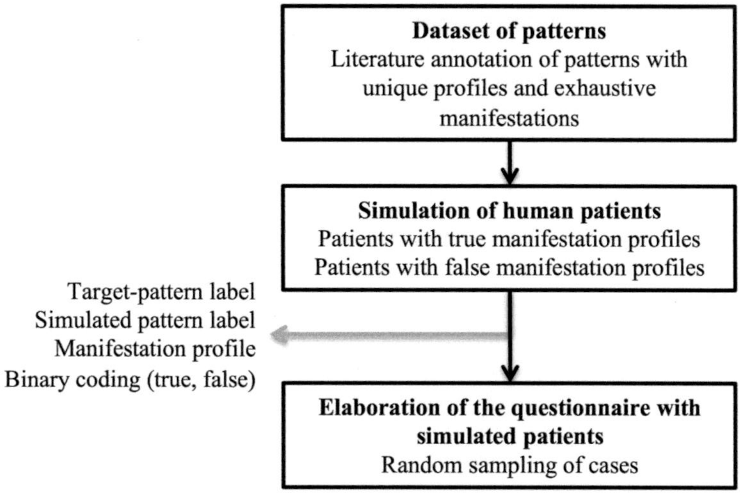

Fig. 7.2 Stages for implementing reliability studies using the framework of simulated patients

identified in previous researchers for that respective disease; whenever this information is not available it is possible to select a set of patterns from CM literature. For instance, a study [23] elaborated a dataset of 73 *zangfu* patterns described by a total of 509 unique manifestations distributed among the four examinations inspection (n = 103, 20.2 %), auscultation-olfaction (n = 31, 6.1 %), inquiry (n = 349, 68.6 %), and palpation (n = 26, 5.1 %). In general, datasets of patterns are made by manual insertion of data from CM literature and thus it is prone to typos and other kinds of errors, such as repeated manifestations within the same pattern. The consistency and quality of the database must be computationally tested before simulation of patients to ensure that patterns are mutually exclusive (i.e., all patters are uniquely described in the dataset) and collectively exhaustive (i.e., all patterns in dataset are related to the underlying disease), and have no duplicated manifestations among the four examinations in each pattern.

7.7.2 *Simulation of Human Patients: True and False Profiles*

The second requirement for simulation of patients is the simulation model itself. As previously explained, the *SimTCM* is a useful model for simulation of patients with respect to CM theory [19, 22]. Briefly, *SimTCM* simulates a patient with a given pattern by selecting variable and random numbers of manifestations that form that pattern. This procedure is repeated for all patterns in the dataset until the desired sample size is achieved. For this simulation, one may assume that the probability for occurring each manifestation for each pattern follows a uniform probability mass function in the general population, or a given probability mass function if available from previous studies. Using the *SimTCM* no user intervention is required other than the set-up of the simulation.

For diagnostic purposes, patients should be simulated under two conditions, namely *true* and *false* profiles; only in this way, contingency tables can be constructed for assessment of diagnostic accuracy. A *true profile* means that *SimTCM* samples a given target-pattern from the dataset, which is actually simulated by sampling manifestations from this same pattern. In this case, the label of the target-pattern equals the label of the simulated one and thus it represents a *case* for that target-pattern. Conversely, a *false profile* means that *SimTCM* samples a given target-pattern from the dataset, excludes it from the dataset, and only then samples another pattern that is actually simulated by sampling manifestations from this another pattern. In this case, the label of the target-pattern differs from the label of the simulated one and thus it represents a *control* for that target-pattern.

These definitions of 'cases' and 'controls' might seem odd at first approach, but it is legit for both CM and epidemiology [39]. From the CM point-of-view to diagnose is to differentiate a pattern among other patterns that are likely to occur and thus an asymptomatic 'control' group for comparison is not adequate. From the epidemiology point-of-view, 'control' groups must include those at risk of presenting such patterns, for instance with the same disease that might present other pattern and not being an asymptomatic subject—although other patterns may be identified in asymptomatic subjects because constitutional, behavioral or emotional characteristics are also of diagnostic value in CM. Nonetheless, both kinds of patients are required if the study aims to access all components of the accuracy, including true- and false-positive, true- and false-negative rates as explained in the upcoming sections.

The following data is exported from *SimTCM* as a combined TXT file to be used in subsequent stages of the research: (i) a label representing the target-pattern under simulation; (ii) a label representing the pattern randomly selected for simulation; (iii) the manifestation profile as comma-separated values; and (iv) the binary code representing the patient as "1" or "0" if the human patient simulated corresponds to either a true profile or a false profile.

7.7.3 Elaboration of the Questionnaire with Simulated Patients

With the sample size of patients calculated and the simulated patients available, the next stage comprises the elaboration of the questionnaire for presentation of such patients to the sample of raters. The sample of simulated patients with known true and false profiles will compose the questionnaire. All questions will be prepared and presented clearly, avoiding dubious interpretation.

To avoid concentration of profiles with the same block of data, i.e., true or false profiles, the questionnaire should be randomly distributed for a better distribution of simulated patients. For this purpose any automated method for generating numbers and sequences can be used, including online resources.[4] Using the R package 'blockrand' [25] is an interesting method for such a task and may begin with the following code:

```
# Install the required package for randomization
require("blockrand")
# Load the package
library(blockrand)
# Display the reference of the package
print(citation(package = "blockrand", lib.loc = NULL))
```

Example Suppose a study protocol simulated 30 patients for generating the questionnaire in a 1:1 ratio of true:false profiles. To create random assignments for an experiment in which the subjects come prospectively, i.e., one at a time (as is the case of the simulated patients to be presented in the questionnaire) the randomization is done within blocks to balance the amount of true and false profiles. By doing this, the ratio of true:false profiles stays close to equal throughout the questionnaire using the following code lines:

```
# Stratified by profile type, 15 in stratum, 2 levels
Q <- blockrand(n=30, num.levels=2, levels=c("True profile", "False profile"), id.prefix="Question #", block.sizes=1:1, uneq.beg=FALSE, uneq.mid=FALSE, uneq.min=0, uneq.maxit=10)
# display the randomization chart
print(Q)
```

which yields a nice balanced randomization of the simulated cases into questions as can be seen in the following output:

[4]Available at www.random.org.

	id	block.id	block.size	Treatment
1	Question #01	1	2	False profile
2	Question #02	1	2	True profile
3	Question #03	2	2	True profile
4	Question #04	2	2	False profile
5	Question #05	3	2	True profile
6	Question #06	3	2	False profile
7	Question #07	4	2	True profile
8	Question #08	4	2	False profile
9	Question #09	5	2	False profile
10	Question #10	5	2	True profile
11	Question #11	6	2	False profile
12	Question #12	6	2	True profile
13	Question #13	7	2	True profile
14	Question #14	7	2	False profile
15	Question #15	8	2	False profile
16	Question #16	8	2	True profile
17	Question #17	9	2	False profile
18	Question #18	9	2	True profile
19	Question #19	10	2	False profile
20	Question #20	10	2	True profile
21	Question #21	11	2	False profile
22	Question #22	11	2	True profile
23	Question #23	12	2	False profile
24	Question #24	12	2	True profile
25	Question #25	13	2	True profile
26	Question #26	13	2	False profile
27	Question #27	14	2	False profile
28	Question #28	14	2	True profile
29	Question #29	15	2	False profile
30	Question #30	15	2	True profile

7.7.4 Face-to-Face Interview of CM Experts Using the Questionnaire

There are several ways for delivering a questionnaire for respondents, including phone calls, printed correspondence, and online surveys. Although online surveys are increasingly used by researchers because of its appealing advantages—including low cost and high coverage of respondents—the quantity of data loss due to missing or incomplete data is also huge. Alternatively, a hardcopy questionnaire may also be delivered face-to-face, containing a brief survey of possible risks and benefits of this research to society and in particular to the respondent. The questionnaire should be self-administered such that the investigator does not interfere in its completion.

The set-up for raters filling-up the questionnaire must be as close as real to the clinical practice. Instead of confining raters into closed laboratories without access to literature, one may consider conducting this stage at the rater's facilities with his/her own literature resources more likely to increase the external validity of the study. To reproduce clinical conditions, the rater may be allowed to consult the reference book used for generating the dataset of patterns, though shall not be encouraged to do so. To the raters, a sufficient amount of time must be allowed to familiarize themselves with the questionnaires and related material; also, no time limit should be posed to complete the questionnaire.

The following material must be available to the rater: a hardcopy table with many options as candidate patterns plus the option "It is not possible to identify the pattern." Likewise, if the reliability for acupuncture prescription is aiming to be assessed a hardcopy table must also be available with many options as candidate acupuncture points (e.g., 361 options for channel acupoints [40], 17 miscellaneous acupoints [4]) plus the option "No acupoint." For questions about the diagnosis, it will be required only one answer; for questions about the acupoints, it might be required 1 or more (up to 8 answers were observed in the literature [9–17]).

A practical strategy is to provide individual, separated response forms for filling the respective answer regarding the identified pattern and the prescribed acupoints for each simulated patient. All these data must be tabulated in electronic worksheets with automatic data validation to avoid typos. If data is typed in Excel (Microsoft Corp., USA) the R package 'xlsx' [31] can be used for data import with the following code lines:

```
# install the required package for import data
require("xlsx")
# load the package
library(xlsx)
# display the reference of the package
print(citation(package = "xlsx", lib.loc = NULL))
# define working directory
local <- setwd(paste(getwd()))
# import data from electronic worksheet
rawdata = as.matrix(read.xlsx("FILENAME.xlsx",
sheetName="SHEETNAME", as.data.frame=TRUE,
header=FALSE, keepFormulas=FALSE))
```

7.8 Data Tabulation for Analysis

The rater's response to each patient must be paired to the numbering of the questions. The coding for responses concerning patterns and acupoints must also be typed into the electronic worksheet, also paired to the numbering of the questions. For calculating reliability for pattern differentiation or acupuncture prescription, the formatting exhibited in Table 7.1 immediately allows the calculation of interrater agreement.

Parameters related to the diagnostic performance [23] of each rater can be obtained from 2 × 2 contingency tables (Table 7.2) made from the comparison between the results of the simulation with *SimTCM* (i.e., gold-standard) and the pattern differentiation by each rater (i.e., diagnostic test result):

- *True-positives* (*TP*): manifestation profiles simulated with the target-pattern that were correctly identified by the rater as present;
- *True-negatives* (*TN*): manifestation profiles not simulated with the target-pattern that were correctly identified by the rater as absent;
- *False-negatives* (*FN*): manifestation profiles simulated with the target-pattern that were erroneously identified by the rater as absent; and
- *False-positives* (*FP*): manifestation profiles not simulated with the target-pattern that were erroneously identified by the rater as present.

7.8.1 Statistical Analysis Plan

Statistical analysis of data is usually separated by study's outcome, including descriptive, comparative, associative, reliability, and diagnostic performance. Herein, a suggestion of statistical analysis plan is provided based on the methods presented.

Table 7.1 Classification table for comparison among n raters assessing N patients

	Rater #				
Patient #	1	2	3	…	n
1	$d_{1,1}$	$d_{1,2}$	$d_{1,3}$	…	$d_{1,n}$
2	$d_{2,1}$	$d_{2,2}$	$d_{2,3}$	…	$d_{2,n}$
3	$d_{3,1}$	$d_{3,2}$	$d_{3,3}$	…	$d_{3,n}$
…	…	…	…	…	…
N	$d_{N,1}$	$d_{N,2}$	$d_{N,3}$	…	$d_{N,n}$

$d_{N,k}$ Categorical datum form each patient as obtained from each rater

7.9 Descriptive

Because of the usually small sample size of raters (5 or less), data analysis must be reported based on single measurements of each rater alongside group values presented as median [minimum; maximum] for continuous variables. Categorical variables must be presented using absolute and relative frequencies (%).

Coefficients of agreement can be qualitatively interpreted as poor (<0.00), slight (0.00–0.20), fair (0.21–0.40), moderate (0.41–0.60), substantial (0.61–0.80), or almost perfect (0.81–1.00) [41].

The correlation values and their qualitative levels of association will be described as no association (0.00), negligible (±0.01 to ±0.20), weak (±0.21 to ±0.40), moderate (±0.41 to ±0.70), strong (±0.71 to ±0.99), or perfect association (±1.00) [42].

7.10 Interrater Agreement of CM Experts for Pattern Differentiation

The Light's κ (kappa) coefficient [43] is recommended for studies with fully crossed design in which all cases are classified by multiple raters [44] for the univariate case (1 variable = the identified pattern).

For a given $n*k$ matrix ('r') with n = sample size of patients and k = sample size of raters), the R package 'psy' [30] presents the command line structure for calculating this statistics:

Table 7.2 Contingency (2 × 2) table for assessment of diagnostic performance of Chinese medicine experts using human patients simulation

		SimTCM output (Reference test)	
		True manifestation profile[a] (Simulated = target)	**False manifestation profile**[b] (Simulated ≠ target)
Result from CM expert (New test)	**Target-pattern** + (Identified = target)	True-positive (*TP*)	False-positive (*FP*)
	Target-pattern − (Identified ≠ target)	False-negative (*FN*)	True-negative (*TN*)
Summary coefficients of diagnostic performance		$SEN = TP/(TP + FN)$	$SPE = TN/(TN + FP)$
		$PPV = TP/(TP + FP)$	$NPV = TN/(TN + FN)$
		$ACC = (TP + TN)/(TP + TN + FP + FN)$	

SEN sensitivity; *SPE* specificity; *PPV* positive predictive value; *NPV* negative predictive value; *ACC* accuracy

[a]Target-pattern present

[b]Target-pattern absent

```
# install the required package for calculation
require("psy")
# load the package
library(psy)
# display the reference of the package
print(citation(package = "psy", lib.loc = NULL))
# general structure
lkappa(r, type = "Cohen", weights = "squared")
```

7.11 Interrater Agreement of CM Experts for Acupuncture Prescription

The κ statistics is only useful for testing reliability for acupuncture prescription in case only one acupoint (i.e., one variable) is expected as a treatment; whenever more than two variables are to be considered simultaneously, the κ coefficient is no longer adequate. The Janson and Olsson's ι (iota) coefficient [45] is recommended for studies with multivariate analysis by multiple raters on the same participants for the multivariate case (N variables = acupoint #1, acupoint #2, …, acupoint #N). Such statistics is an estimate corrected for chance agreement in multivariate classifications from several raters. Statistics ι is interpreted as an extension of κ for several raters and several variables.

For a given list ('ratings') of k matrices sized $n*m$ with one list element for each variable, n = sample size of patients, and k = sample size of raters the R package 'irr' [28] presents the command lines for calculating this statistics as follows:

```
# install the required package for calculation
require("irr")
# load the package
library(irr)
# display the reference of the package
print(citation(package = "irr", lib.loc = NULL))
# general structure
iota(ratings, scaledata= c("quantitative", "nominal"),
standardize=FALSE)
```

7.12 Diagnostic Performance of CM Experts

Accuracy (*ACC*), sensitivity (*SEN*), positive predictive value (*PPV*), specificity (*SPE*), and negative predictive values (*NPV*) can be calculated according to the equations in Table 7.2 [46, 47]. Results from both single rating and whole sample rating using the output from *SimTCM* as gold-standard and the output from CM raters must be provided separately.

The R package 'caret' [27] presents the command lines for calculating this statistics as follows:

```
# install the required package for analysis of confusion
matrix
require("caret")
# load the package
library(caret)
# display the reference of the package
print(citation(package = "caret", lib.loc = NULL))
# calculating coefficients from confusion matrix
confusionMatrix(data, reference, positive=NULL, dnn= c
("Prediction", "Reference"), prevalence=NULL)
```

7.13 Associative Analysis

The researcher might be interested in investigation the relationship between the personal characteristics of the sample of raters and the diagnostic performance for pattern differentiation. This finding may be observed using the Spearman's ρ correlation coefficient [48] by analyzing the correlation of control with outcome variables. The Spearman correlation is the method of choice because both the small sample sizes of raters and the measurement scale of the variables to be tested for association.

7.14 Confidence Intervals

Confidence intervals [95 %CI] might be calculated using the bootstrap procedure and bias-corrected accelerated method (BCa) using the R package 'boot' [29], with $B = 1000$ replications [49]. Empirical p values might be calculated from the 95 % CI using $(r + 1)/(B + 1)$, where r is the number of replications that produce p values greater than or equal to the p value calculated with statistical data [50].

7.15 Concluding Remarks

This chapter presented and discussed methodological choices for designing study protocols aiming to investigate interrater reliability for pattern differentiation and acupoint prescription. Developing a study protocol for unveiling these outcomes is particularly challenging: to combine traditional theories with contemporary instruments and procedures without mutual interference is virtually impossible.

Particularly, the major challenge comprised the need of a gold-standard method for assessing the accuracy of pattern differentiation and the presentation of these cases to the CM experts in a systematic fashion. We recommend to use patients simulation instead of real cases, and consequently to present them as a written list of manifestations. Although this methodological choice provides a gold-standard method for measuring accuracy, it might compromise the observation of clinically meaningful information for pattern differentiation. As a corollary, diagnostic accuracy itself may be underestimated as compared to real human patients from whom additional data can be obtained during the interview. Nonetheless, the use of written clinical cases has been the method of knowledge transmission regarding CM for at least two millennia and thus it is consistent with the CM's mode of thinking. Because face-to-face interviews have been considered as the approach of choice for data collection in epidemiological studies, questionnaire becomes an important tool in the study of diagnostic accuracy when combined with robust software for data simulation and analyzing the responses of CM experts.

From the methodological point of view, study protocol designed with more robust methods also highlights new methodologies to the CM field, which are already available in epidemiology, statistics and related areas. The usage of separated coefficients of agreement for the univariate (pattern differentiation $\rightarrow \kappa$) and multivariate problems (acupunctures prescription $\rightarrow \iota$) comprises a novelty in comparison to the previous ones on this subject. The majority of the previous studies used simple percent agreement for assessing reliability, which is not recommended mainly because it is not chance-corrected. Although both κ and ι have their own limitations, they possess desirable characteristics for coefficients of agreement and are applicable to CM problems as well.

The Chinese art of pattern differentiation for diagnosis is essentially a subjective analysis. Therefore, the quantification and standardization of diagnostic procedures for CM practitioners are an urgent need. The last two decades have witnessed the growth of importance of research related to computerization of pattern differentiation. Important advances in biomedical instrumentation and software development opened new possibilities to research on this important aspect regarding CM examination. Therefore, planning research studies with an integrative design is a unique challenge but is also a required step towards the development of an evidence-based practice of CM. It is expected that the information herein might provide new insights about interrater reliability for diagnosis and intervention.

Acknowledgments This work was supported by a grant from the Fundação Carlos Chagas Filho de Amparo à Pesquisa do Estado do Rio de Janeiro.

References

1. World Health Organization. Primary Health Care Report of the International Conference on Primary Health Care, Alma-Ata, USSR, 6–12 Sept 1978. Geneva, 1978.
2. T'ao L. Chinese medicine during the Chin (1127–1234) and Yuan (1234–1368) eras. Chin Med J. 1955;73(3):241–56.
3. Lee T, Cheng CF, Chang CS. Some early records of nervous and mental diseases in traditional Chinese medicine. Chin Med J. 1962;81:55–9.
4. O'Connor J, Bensky D. Acupuncture a comprehensive text. Seattle: Eastland Press; 1987.
5. Ferreira AS, Lopes AJ. Chinese medicine pattern differentiation and its implications for clinical practice. Chin J Integr Med. 2011;17(11):818–23.
6. Weingart SN, Wilson RM, Gibberd RW, Harrison B. Epidemiology of medical error. Br Med J. 2000;320(18):774–7.
7. Kuhn GJ. Diagnostic errors. Acad Emerg Med. 2002;9(7):740–50.
8. Schiff GD, Hasan O, Kim S, Abrams R, Cosby R, Lambert BL, Elstein AS, Hasler S, Kabongo ML, Krosnjar N, Odwazny R, Wisniewski MF, McNutt RA. Diagnostic errors in medicine: analysis of 583 physician-reported errors. Arch Int Med. 2009;169(20):1881–7.
9. Sung JJY, Leung WK, Ching JYL, Lao L, Zhang G, Wu JCY, Liang SM, Xie H, Ho YP, Chan LS, Bernam B, Chan FKL. Agreements among traditional Chinese medicine practitioners in the diagnosis and treatment of irritable bowel syndrome. Aliment Pharmacol Ther. 2004;20(10):1205–10.
10. Zhang GG, Lee W, Bausell B, Lao L, Handwerger B, Berman B. Variability in the traditional Chinese medicine (TCM) diagnoses and herbal prescriptions provided by three TCM practitioners for 40 patients with rheumatoid arthritis. J Altern Complement Med. 2005; 11(3):415–21.
11. Zhang GG, Singh B, Lee W, Handwerger B, Lao L, Berman B. Improvement of agreement in TCM diagnosis among TCM practitioners for persons with the conventional diagnosis of rheumatoid arthritis: effect of training. J Altern Complement Med. 2008;14(4):381–6.
12. Coyetaux RR, Chen W, Lindemuth CE, Tan Y, Reilly AC. Variability in the diagnosis and point selection for persons with frequent headache by traditional Chinese medicine acupuncturists. J Altern Complement Med. 2006;12(9):863–72.
13. Mist S, Ritenbaugh C, Aickin M. Effects of questionnaire-based diagnosis and training on inter-rater reliability among practitioners of traditional Chinese medicine. J Altern Complement Med. 2009;15(7):703–9.
14. O'Brien KA, Abbas E, Zhang J, Guo Z, Luo R, Bensoussan A, Komesaroff PA. An investigation into the reliability of Chinese medicine diagnosis according to the eight guiding principles and Zang-fu theory in Australians with hypercholesterolemia. J Altern Complement Med. 2009;15(3):259–66.
15. Grant SJ, Schnyer RN, Chang DH, Fahey P, Bensoussan A. Interrater reliability of Chinese medicine diagnosis in people with prediabetes. Evid Based Complem Altern Med. 2013;2013: Article ID 710892.
16. Birkeflet O, Laake P, Vollestad NK. Poor multi-rater reliability in TCM pattern diagnoses and variation in the use of symptoms to obtain a diagnosis. Acupunct Med. 2014;32(4):325–32.
17. Xu ZX, Xu J, Yan JJ, Wang YQ, Guo R, Liu GP, Yan HX, Qian P, Hong YJ. Analysis of the diagnostic consistency of Chinese medicine specialists in cardiovascular disease cases and syndrome identification based on the relevant feature for each label learning method. Chin J Integr Med. (30 Jul 2014, Epub ahead of print).

18. Ferreira AS. Advances in Chinese medicine diagnosis: from traditional methods to computational models. In: Kuang H, editor. Recent advances in Chinese medicine. Croatia: InTech; 2012.
19. Ferreira AS. Promoting the Integrative Medicine by the computerization of traditional Chinese medicine for scientific research and clinical practice: The SuiteTCM Project. J Integr Med. 2013;11(2):135–9.
20. Ferreira AS, Pacheco AG. SimTCM: a human patient simulator with application to diagnostic accuracy studies of Chinese medicine. J Integr Med. (Dec 2014, Epub ahead of print).
21. de Sá Ferreira A. Statistical validation of strategies for Zang-fu single pattern differentiation. J Chin Integr Med. 2008;6(11):1109–16.
22. Ferreira AS. Diagnostic accuracy of pattern differentiation algorithm based on traditional Chinese medicine theory: a stochastic simulation study. Chin Med. 2009;4:24.
23. Sá Ferreira A. Misdiagnosis and undiagnosis due to pattern similarity in Chinese medicine: a stochastic simulation study using pattern differentiation algorithm. Chin Med. 2011;6:13.
24. R Core Team. R: a language and environment for statistical computing. Vienna, Austria: R Foundation for Statistical Computing.
25. Snow G. blockrand: Randomization for block random clinical trials. 2013. R package version 1.3.
26. Canty A, Ripley B. boot: Bootstrap R (S-Plus) functions. 2014. R package version 1.3-11.
27. Kuhn M. Contributions from Jed Wing, Steve Weston, Andre Williams, Chris Keefer, Allan Engelhardt, Tony Cooper, Zachary Mayer, Brenton Kenkel, the R Core Team and Michael Benesty. caret: Classification and Regression Training. 2014. R package version 6.0-37.
28. Gamer M, Lemon J, Singh IFP. irr: Various Coefficients of Interrater Reliability and Agreement. 2012. R package version 0.84.
29. Rotondi MA. kappaSize: Sample Size Estimation Functions for Studies of Interobserver Agreement. 2013. R package version 1.1.
30. Falissard B. psy: Various procedures used in psychometry. 2012. R package version 1.1.
31. Dragulescu AA. xlsx: Read, write, format Excel 2007 and Excel 97/2000/XP/2003 files. 2014. R package version 0.5.7.
32. Kottner J, Audigé L, Brorson S, Donner A, Gajewski BJ, Hróbjartsson A, Roberts C, Shoukri M, Streiner DL. Guidelines for Reporting Reliability and Agreement Studies (GRRAS) were proposed. J Clin Epidemiol. 2011;64(1):96–106.
33. MacPherson H, Altman DG, Hammerschlag R, Youping L, Taixing W, White A, Moher D, STRICTA Revision Group. Revised STandards for Reporting Interventions in Clinical Trials of Acupuncture (STRICTA): extending the CONSORT statement. PLoS Med. 2010;7(6): e1000261.
34. MacPherson H, White A, Cummings M, Jobst K, Rose K, Niemtzow R. Standards for reporting interventions in controlled trials of acupuncture: The STRICTA recommendations. STandards for Reporting Interventions in Controlled Trails of Acupuncture. Acupunct Med. 2002;20(1):22–5.
35. Bossuyt PM, Reitsma JB, Bruns DE, Gatsonis CA, Glasziou PP, Irwig LM, Moher D, Rennie D, de Vet HCW, Lijmer JG. The STARD statement for reporting studies of diagnostic accuracy: explanation and elaboration. Ann Intern Med. 2003;138:W1–2.
36. Altaye M, Donner A, Eliasziw M. A general goodness-of-fit approach for inference procedures concerning the kappa statistic. Stat Med. 2011;20(16):2479–88.
37. Siemiatycki J, Campbell S. Nonresponse bias and early versus all responders in mail and telephone surveys. Am J Epidemiol. 1984;120(2):291–301.
38. Shin BC, Kim S, Cho YH. Syndrome pattern and its application in parallel randomized controlled trials. Chin J Integr Med. 2013;19(3):163–71.
39. Grimes DA, Schulz KF. Compared to what? Finding controls for case-control studies. Lancet. 2005;365:1429–33.
40. World Health Organization. Standard acupuncture nomenclature. Geneva: World Health Organization; 1993.

41. Landis JR, Koch GG. The measurement of observer agreement for categorical data. Biometrics. 1977;33(1):159–74.
42. World Health Organization. Health research methodology: a guide for training in research methods. Geneva: World Health Organization; 2001.
43. Light RJ. Measures of response agreement for qualitative data: some generalizations and alternatives. Psychol Bull. 1971;76(5):365–77.
44. Hallgren KA. Computing inter-rater reliability for observational data: an overview and tutorial. Tutor Quant Methods Psychol. 2012;8(1):23–34.
45. Janson H, Olsson U. A measure of agreement for interval or nominal multivariate observations. Educ Psychol Measur. 2001;6(21):277–89.
46. Altman DG, Bland JM. Diagnostic tests. 1: Sensitivity and specificity. BMJ. 1994;308 (6943):1552.
47. Altman DG, Bland JM. Diagnostic tests 2: Predictive values. BMJ. 1994;309(6947):102.
48. Kanji G. 100 statistical tests. 3a edição. London: Sage Publications; 2006.
49. Efron B, Tibshirani RJ. An introduction to the bootstrap. Florida: CRC Press; 1998.
50. North BV, Curtis D, Sham PC. A note on the calculation of empirical P-values from Monte Carlo procedures. Am J Hum Genet. 2002;71(2):439–41.

Chapter 8
Bioinformatics for Molecular Authentication of Chinese Medicinal Materials

Ka-Lok Wong, Yat-Tung Lo and Pang-Chui Shaw

Abstract Correctly identified medicinal materials are the premise of research and applications on Chinese medicine. DNA authentication is an accurate method for routine identification of medicinal herbs. The molecular authentication procedure involving DNA sequencing takes five steps: (a) to extract DNA from the sample, (b) to amplify a specific region of the genome by polymerase chain reaction; (c) to sequence the PCR product; (d) to find the available DNA sequences in a nucleotide database; and (e) to compare the unknown sequence with the available reference sequences. Molecular authentication can also be done by DNA fingerprinting that assess the whole or specific region of genome. In the process, informatics assists in: (a) providing a means for storing, sorting, retrieving, and analyzing of experimental data; (b) providing computer programs for identifying the unknown sample by matching with the reference sequences; and (c) aiding the design of appropriate testing procedures and identification tools. This chapter introduces several public databases for the search of taxonomic and nucleotide information, such as Flora of China, NCBI Nucleotide database, Barcode of Life Data Systems (BOLD), and Medicinal Materials DNA Barcode Database (MMDBD). The procedures of mass retrieving and sorting of sequences from databases will be demonstrated. The pros and cons of various DNA sequence formats like FASTA, Abstract Syntax Notation 1 (ASN1), eXtensible Markup Language (XML) will be discussed. Finally, the precautions of using software packages for performing sequence alignment, matching species in databases, and constructing phylogenetic trees will be described.

Ka-Lok Wong and Yat-Tung Lo: Equal contribution.

K.-L. Wong (✉) · Y.-T. Lo (✉) · P.-C. Shaw
State Key Laboratory of Phytochemistry and Plant Resources in West China (CUHK), LDS YYC R&D Centre for Chinese Medicine, School of Life Sciences, The Chinese University of Hong Kong, Hong Kong, China
e-mail: klwong@cuhk.edu.hk

Y.-T. Lo
e-mail: ytlo@cuhk.edu.hk

P.-C. Shaw
e-mail: pcshaw@cuhk.edu.hk

S. Leung and H. Hu (eds.), *Evidence-based Research Methods for Chinese Medicine*, DOI 10.1007/978-981-10-2290-6_8

Keywords Chinese medicinal materials · Authentication · Bioinformatics · DNA

8.1 Introduction

Bioinformatics is an interdisciplinary science, utilizing various informatics techniques, such as computer sciences, statistics ,and mathematics to analyze, organize, and understand biological data, especially nucleotide and protein sequences [1]. The term Bioinformatics was first coined by Paulien Hogeweg and Ben Hesper in 1978 [2] which was defined as "a study of information transfer in biological system," but after 1980, it was changed to "conceptualizing biology of macromolecules information" [3]. Since the publication of the double-helix model of DNA structure in 1953 [4] and the first complete genome sequencing of bacteria in the 1995 [5], numerous genomic data have been available thereafter. In order to deal with and share such great amount of information, biological databases have been established which act as platforms for data storage, analyzes and exchange. With the advance of internet technologies, some online databases and software programs are accessible that further reduce cost and time. Nowadays, bioinformatics is an indispensable part of biomedical and life sciences research. It also becomes a conventional tool for molecular authentication of Chinese medicinal materials. In the 2010 edition of Pharmacopeia of the People's Republic of China (PPRC), molecular techniques have first been announced as a legal basis for the authentication of Chinese medicine materials, including Agkistrodon (Qishe), Fritillariae Cirrhosae Bulbus (Chuanbeimu), and Zaocys (Wushaoshe) [6]. There are two general approaches for molecular authentication of Chinese medicinal materials: generating DNA fingerprints and DNA sequencing. In this chapter, we put more emphasis on the bioinformatics of DNA sequencing, as it is a more definitive method.

8.2 The Role of Bioinformatics in Molecular Authentication

Bioinformatics has three major roles in molecular authentication: (a) to provide a mean for storing, sorting, retrieving, and analyzing of experimental data. There are about 900 species recorded in PPRC [6], of which DNA sequences of over 700 species have already been recorded in the Nucleotide databases of National Center for Biotechnology Information (NCBI) [7]. The Medicinal Materials DNA Barcode Database (MMDBD, http://www.cuhk.edu.hk/icm/mmdbd.htm) developed by our group has also recorded 1661 species of medicinal herbal sequences and their adulterants [8]; (b) to provide computer programs for identifying an unknown sample by matching its sequence with the database sequences. In principle, genome sequence of a species is unique, and therefore, it can be used for identification purpose. Even the reference sequence is not available, one is often able to find a related sequence and obtain the identity at genera level. Phylogenetic tree can also be constructed to understand the evolutionary relationship between related herbal species, which may aid for finding alternative; and (c) to aid the design of appropriate testing procedures and identification tools in DNA fingerprinting, DNA sequencing, and DNA microarray. In principle, mutations in DNA sequences, like substitution, insertion, deletion, duplication, and even single nucleotide polymorphism (SNP) are markers for species identification. Bioinformatics tools help to search, process, and utilize these sites from massive amount of data.

8.3 Workflow of Molecular Authentication

The process of molecular authentication on medicinal materials generally involves three major steps: extracting DNA from medicinal materials, amplification of DNA loci, and data analysis. Besides DNA extraction, subsampling from different batches or positions of the sample is also important for consistent identification results (Sect. 8.4).

To find the identity of an unknown sample, DNA barcoding, which is based on determining a short genetic sequence from the standard part of genome with species differentiation power [9], is often employed (Sect. 8.5). Basic local alignment search tool (BLAST) is then performed to check the quality of generated sequence and to get a preliminary identification (Sect. 8.8.1). The identity of the unknown sample is further validated using Clustal (Sect. 8.8.2) by comparing sample sequence with reference sequences, in many cases, downloaded from databases (Sect. 8.7). Analyzing programs are then employed to calculate the sequence similarities (Sect. 8.9.1) and construct phylogenetic trees to reveal the relationship among the identified samples and its related species (Sect. 8.9.2) (Fig. 8.1).

Another molecular authentication approach is DNA fingerprinting. This approach is simpler and quicker than DNA sequencing but less definitive. It can be subdivided into whole genome and specific region approaches and are briefly described in Sects. 8.10.1 and 8.10.2, respectively. To design a diagnostic primer for specific region DNA fingerprinting, the taxonomic information of the target species, its closely related species and common adulterants should be obtained from databases for organism classification and nomenclature (Sect. 8.6) with a view to defining the scope of the test. DNA sequences are then downloaded from nucleotide databases (Sect. 8.7) and aligned (Sect. 8.8.2) for primer design (Sect. 8.10.2.1) or using NEBCutter to find available restriction sites (Sect. 8.10.2.2). They have to be experimentally validated (Fig. 8.2).

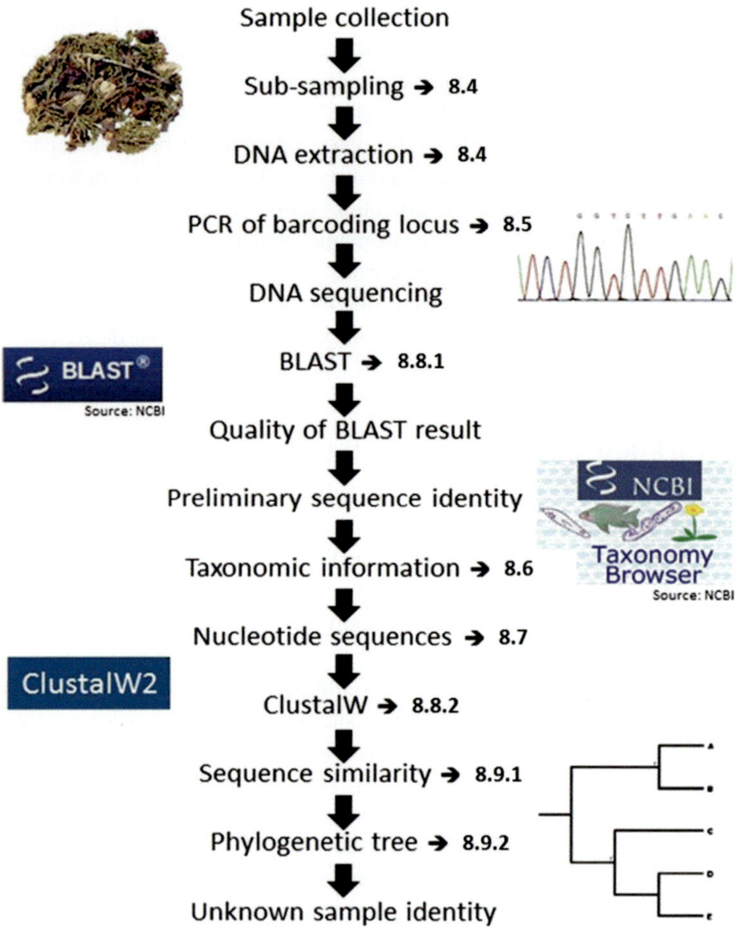

Fig. 8.1 Overview of the steps involved in identifying unknown samples using DNA barcoding techniques. *Number* indicates the section at which the topic is discussed

8.4 Sampling, DNA Extraction and Purification

It is advisable to collect and test more than one sample from the same batch of medicinal materials. Sampling from solid materials should be taken from the top, middle, and bottom sections; while liquid materials should be taken after careful homogenization [6, 10]. Obtaining high quantity and quality of DNA is also crucial for molecular authentication because many polymerase chain reaction (PCR)-based methods are sensitive to DNA degradation [11] and inhibitors [12]. Several extraction protocols are commonly used: potassium acetate/sodium dodecyl sulfate (SDS) [13], cetyltrimethylammonium bromide (CTAB) [14] and "ready-to-use" kits. The first method is suitable for most medicinal materials while CTAB

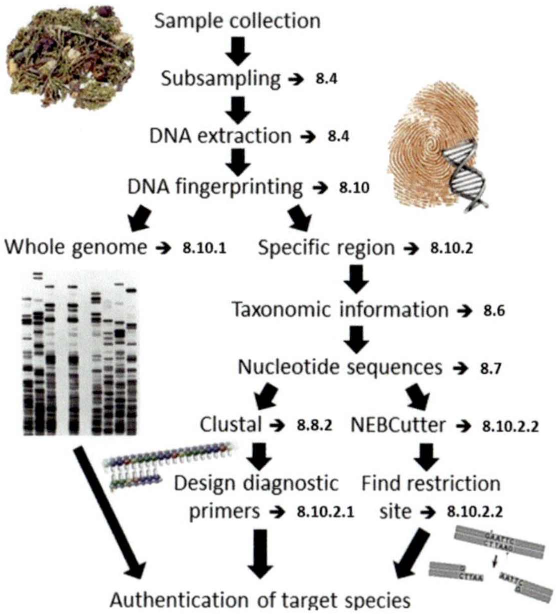

Fig. 8.2 Overview of the steps involved in identifying unknown samples using DNA fingerprinting. *Number* indicates the section at which the topic is discussed

extraction especially suitable for most plants and their treated samples [15]. "Ready-to-use" kits provide a convenient means of extracting high-quality DNA. The extraction procedure usually involves: (i) mechanical breakthrough and solubilize cell membrane to release nucleic acid into solution, (ii) removal of solid residue in high salt solution, so that nucleic acids do not electrostatically bind to it, (iii) binding of nucleic acid to the silica matrix with contaminants flowing thorough the column by centrifugation, and (iv) elution of concentrated DNA from the matrix for analysis [16]. In order to assess the quantity and quality of DNA extracted, measurement of UV absorbance at 260 and 280 nm is recommended. The 260/280 nm ratio of DNA at 1.8 or above is generally regarded as pure. If this ratio is lower than 1.8, it may probably due to the presence of protein, phenol or other contaminants which have a strong absorbance at 280 nm. 260/230 nm is another indicator of nucleic acid purity and it should commonly in the range of 2.0–2.2 [17].

8.5 DNA Barcoding

In 2003, Paul Hebert and colleagues proposed the use of DNA barcodes for species identification purpose [9]. DNA barcodes possess the following features: (a) primer binding sites are conserved across different groups of organisms, (b) easy to be amplified with a single primer pair, (c) highly polymorphic interspecifically but (d) low in intraspecific variation. For instance, the mitochondrial cytochrome c oxidase subunit I (*COI*) gene is suggested as barcode for animal and other eukaryotes [9]; chloroplast large subunit of the ribulose-bisphosphate carboxylase gene (*rbcL*) and maturase K (*matK*) genes are selected for land plants [18]; and nuclear internal transcribed spacer (ITS) region are designated for fungi [19].

8.6 Databases for Organism Classification and Nomenclature

The diversity of medicinal materials is extraordinary: majorly plants, with numerous animals and fungi. Besides the herbs listed in PPRC, it is estimated that there are about ten thousand of organisms currently used as ethnic drugs [20]. Databases of organism classification and nomenclature hold and organize information regarding biological taxa. NCBI (http://www.ncbi.nlm.nih.gov) is a platform provides the access of living organism information. Taxonomy database of NCBI (http://www.ncbi.nlm.nih.gov/taxonomy) is a classification and nomenclature domain for all of the organisms in public sequence database. As Taxonomy and Nucleotide of NCBI are interconnected, relevant nucleotide data of a taxon can be retrieved via the hyperlink. Flora of China (http://flora.huh.harvard.edu/china) is an authoritative document in Chinese plant taxonomy [21], and it describes more than 30,000 kinds of plants for their nomenclatures, morphologies, habitats, geographical distribution, and economic values. The International Plant Names Index (IPNI, http://www.ipni.org), Tropicos (http://www.tropicos.org) and Index Nominum Genericorum (ING, http://botany.si.edu/ing/) are online database of the names and associated basic bibliographical details of plant worldwide. Medicinal Plant Names Services (MPNS, http://mpns.kew.org/mpns-portal) provides pharmaceutical, trade and common names besides taxonomy, and scientific nomenclature of medicinal plants and herbal materials. In addition, our group has established the first database for DNA barcoding of Chinese medicinal materials: MMDBD. Besides various DNA sequences, it provides photos and description of the herbs and online searching and comparison services [8].

The role of database for organism classification and nomenclature in molecular authentication is to define the scope and range of species to be studied. For instance, for designing diagnostic primers to differentiate ginseng (*Panax ginseng*) from its closely related species, researchers should consult Flora of China, MPNS or other databases to obtain the list of species in genus *Panax*. Taxonomy database of NCBI also acts as a starting point for the retrieval of nucleotide sequences. One downloading approach is to first get the target scopes of species in this Taxonomy database, and the result page gives the lineage and ranks (order, family, genus, etc.) of the species. Using the identification of *P. ginseng* as an example again, searching this species in Taxonomy database will generate hyperlinks for each rank. To get the information of all species in *Panax*, user can click hyperlink “Panax.” If test needs to identify all species in family Araliaceae (the family that *P. ginseng* belongs to), just click the hyperlink “Araliaceae” (Fig. 8.3). For the sequence downloading procedures in NCBI, please refer to Sect. 8.7.

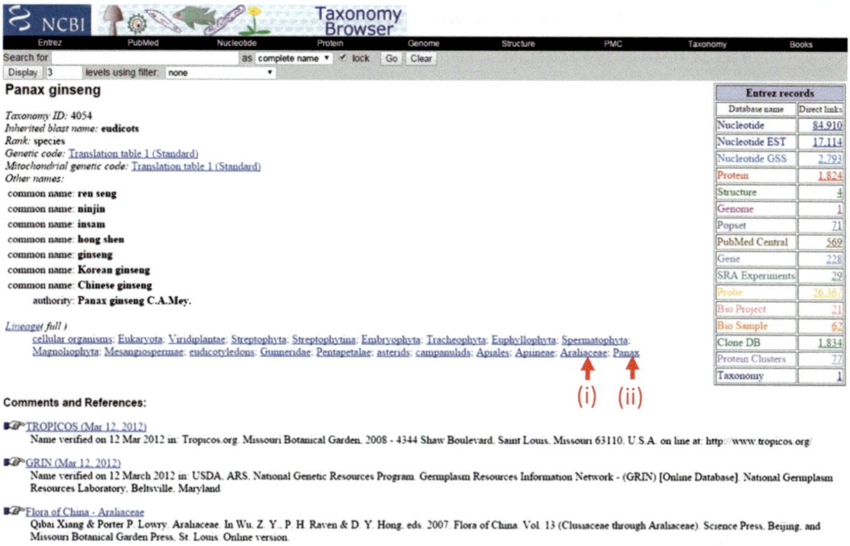
NCBI
Taxonomy Browser
Entrez PubMed Nucleotide Protein Genome Structure PMC Taxonomy Books
Search for as complete name lock Go Clear
Display 3 levels using filter: none
Panax ginseng
Taxonomy ID: 4054
Inherited blast name: eudicots
Rank: species
Genetic code: Translation table 1 (Standard)
Mitochondrial genetic code: Translation table 1 (Standard)
Other names:
common name: ren seng
common name: ninjin
common name: insam
common name: hong shen
common name: ginseng
common name: Korean ginseng
common name: Chinese ginseng
authority: Panax ginseng C.A.Mey.
Lineage(full)
cellular organisms; Eukaryota; Viridiplantae; Streptophyta; Streptophytina; Embryophyta; Tracheophyta; Euphyllophyta; Spermatophyta; Magnoliophyta; Mesangiospermae; eudicotyledons; Gunneridae; Pentapetalae; asterids; campanulids; Apiales; Apiineae; Araliaceae; Panax
(i) (ii)
Entrez records
Database name Direct links
Nucleotide 84,910
Nucleotide EST 17,114
Nucleotide GSS 2,793
Protein 1,824
Structure 4
Genome 1
Popset 71
PubMed Central 569
Gene 228
SRA Experiments 29
Probe 26,367
Bio Project 21
Bio Sample 62
Clone DB 1,834
Protein Clusters 77
Taxonomy 1
Comments and References:
TROPICOS (Mar 12, 2012)
Name verified on 12 Mar 2012 in: Tropicos.org. Missouri Botanical Garden. 2008 - 4344 Shaw Boulevard. Saint Louis, Missouri 63110. U.S.A. on line at: http://www.tropicos.org/
GRIN (Mar 12, 2012)
Name verified on 12 March 2012 in: USDA, ARS, National Genetic Resources Program. Germplasm Resources Information Network - (GRIN) [Online Database]. National Germplasm Resources Laboratory, Beltsville, Maryland
Flora of China - Araliaceae
Qibai Xiang & Porter P. Lowry. Araliaceae. In Wu, Z. Y., P. H. Raven & D. Y. Hong, eds. 2007. Flora of China. Vol. 13 (Clusiaceae through Araliaceae). Science Press, Beijing, and Missouri Botanical Garden Press, St. Louis. Online version.

Fig. 8.3 Search page of NCBI Taxonomy databases. After taxonomic search, NCBI Taxonomy database will show a summary of the target species, including its common names, lineage and Entrez records held in other NCBI databases. User can retrieve the relevant information of each rank via the hyperlinks, for example, (*i*) Family Araliaceae and (*ii*) Genus *Panax*

8.7 Databases of Nucleotide Information

Nucleotide database is a core part of bioinformatics. In DNA barcoding, nucleotide database provides standard sequences as markers for species identification. Moreover, the nucleotide sequences are prerequisite of diagnostic primer design (Sect. 8.10.2.1) which is implemented by finding sequence differences between genuine species and its adulterant (Sect. 8.9). International Nucleotide Sequence Database Collaboration (INSDC, http://insdc.org) comprises GenBank of NCBI, the European Molecular Biology Laboratory (EMBL) [22] and DNA Databank of Japan (DDBJ) [23]. These three organizations exchange data on a daily basis. The Nucleotide database (http://www.ncbi.nlm.nih.gov/nuccore) of NCBI is a collection of sequences from several sources, including GenBank. The Barcode of Life Data Systems (BOLD, http://www.boldsystems.org) is an online database for acquisition, storage, analysis, and publication of DNA barcode sequences [24], which also allows barcoding sequences accession and facilitates species identification by simply matching the unknown sample sequences with the reference barcoding sequences in the databases. Following is the guideline for obtaining the nucleotide sequences from the NCBI Nucleotide database.

8.7.1 Acquisition of Nucleotide Information from NCBI Nucleotide Database

NCBI Nucleotide database accepts sequence data submission from research groups. Like NCBI Taxonomy database, Nucleotide database is cross-platform in nature which allows users to get quick access and track for the related information. In practice, users can directly use the locus name, such as "internal transcribed spacer 2," as a query. To make the search more specific, include the Boolean operators AND, OR, NOT between keywords. The query of "(Panax ginseng) AND (internal transcribed spacer 2)" can retrieve all ITS2 sequences of *P. ginseng* from the database system. "Nucleotide Advanced Search Builder" is a user interface that facilitates building search criteria without memorizing complex syntax (Fig. 8.4a). After searching, Nucleotide database will show a summary of matched sequence entries. User can alter the display format, the number of records shown on each page, and the sort order, by choosing different options within "Display Settings" drop down menu at the left-hand corner. Information can be exported in several formats, including FASTA, Abstract Syntax Notation One (ASN.1) and three types of XML files (Sect. 8.7.2), by clicking "Send to" drop down menu at the right hand corner (Fig. 8.4b).

8.7.2 Sequence Format

FASTA is originally the name of a sequence alignment software package. The file format gradually becomes a standard due to the widely acceptance of FASTA in the field of life sciences. Each sequence in FASTA format has two parts: a description line that starts with ">" symbol followed by the identifier of the sequence, and lines of sequences data (Fig. 8.5). The majority of sequence analyzing program accepts FASTA format, including BLAST [25] (Sect. 8.8.1), Clustal [26] (Sect. 8.8.2), Muscle [27], and BioEdit [28]. Although FASTA is versatile, compact and cross-platform, except for the identifier and sequence, it carries limited background information of the sequence. NCBI offers ASN.1, an International Standards Organization (ISO) data representation format, as an alternative to FASTA. NCBI uses ASN.1 for the storage and retrieval of nucleotide data and consequentially the downloaded ASN.1 file contains all the information of the sequence. Scripting languages like Pearl can parse ASN.1 to extract required data fields. Recently, NCBI gives eXtensible Markup Language (XML) as another option. XML is a markup language that defines rule for encoding documents, and it becomes the standard for online data exchange [29]. Extensible Stylesheet Language Transformations (XSLT) is used to transform the tags and data in the XML file into other formats. To draw an analogy, the tags and data in XML like the alphabets, and XSLT likes the spelling. By using different XSLT files, user can obtain the desired

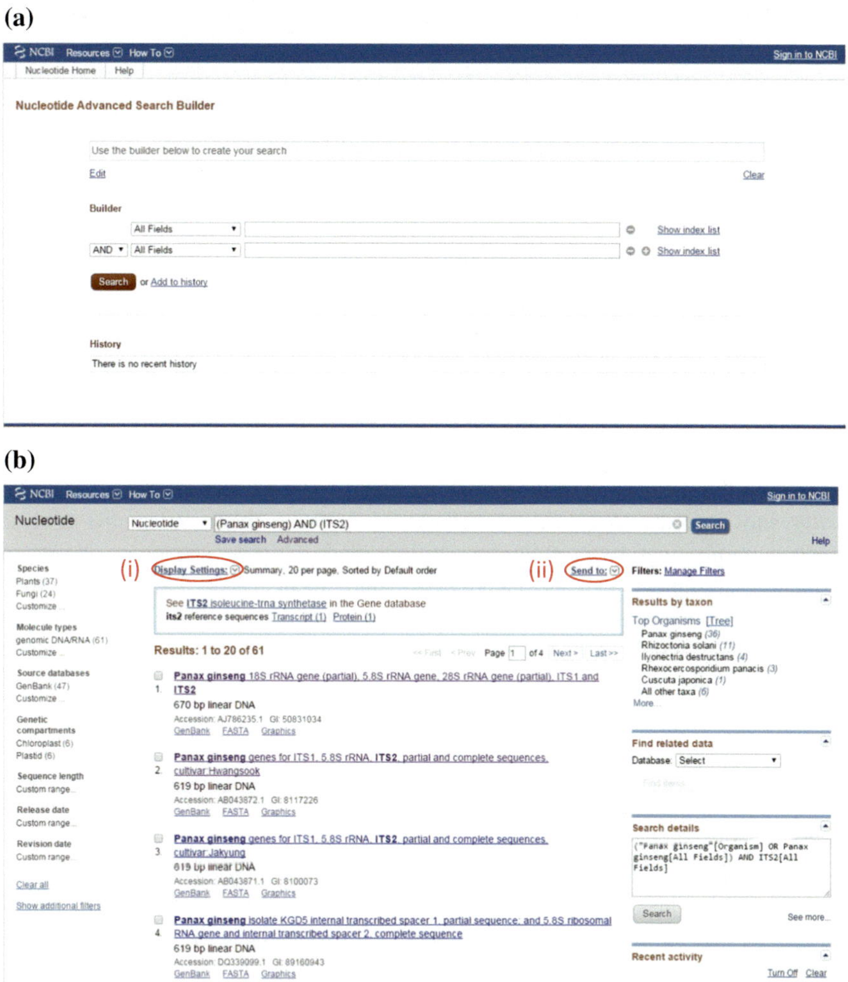

Fig. 8.4 Search page of NCBI Nucleotide database. **a** NCBI Nucleotide database provides a "Nucleotide Advanced Search Builder" function which allows user to combine words and phrases to define the searching parameters. **b** After searching, nucleotide database will show a summary of matched sequence entries. (*i*) User can alter the display format, the number of records shown on each page and the sort order, by choosing different options within "Display Settings" drop down menu. (*ii*) Information can be exported in several formats by clicking "Send to" drop down menu

information (spell the vocabulary) using the same XML file (the alphabets). NCBI distributes three kinds of XML formats, including XML, INSDSeq XML and TinySeq XML. Since the simple data structure of TinySeq XML, Microsoft Excel can directly convert and open it. XML and INSDSeq XML are much complicated and a custom XSLT is required for the transformation.

```
>gi|50831034|emb|AJ786235.1| Panax ginseng 18S rRNA gene (partial), 5.8S rRNA gene, 28S
rRNA gene (partial), ITS1 and ITS2
CGTAGGTGAACCTGCGGAAGGATCATTGTCGAAACCTGCATAGCAGAACGACCCGCGAACACGTTACAAT
ACCGGGTGAGGGACGAGGGGTGCGCAAGCTCCCCAAGTTGCAAACCCATGGTCGGGGACCACCCTTGGGT
GGATCTCGTCCGAACAACGACCCCCCGGCGCGGAATGCGCCAAGGAAATCAAACTGAACTGCACGCGTCC
CCCCCGTTTGCGGGCGGCGGAAGCGTCTTTCTAAAACACAAACGACTCTCGACAACGGATATCTCGGCTC
TCGCATCGATGAAGAACGTAGCGAAATGCGATACTTGGTGTGAATTGCAGAATCCCGTGAACCATCGAGT
CTTTGAACGCAAGTTGCGCCCGAAGCCATTAGGCCGAGGGCACGTCTGCCTGGGCGTCACGCATCGCGTC
GCCCCCCAACCCATCACTCCCTTGCGGGAGTTGAGGCGGAGGGGCGGATAATGGCCTCCCGTGTCTCACC
GCGCGGTTGGCCCAAATGCGAGTCCTTGGCGATGGACGTCACGACAAGTGGTGGTTGTAAAAAGCCCTCT
TCTCATGTCGTGCGGTGACCCGTCGCCAGCAAAAGCTCTCATGACCCTGTTGCGCCGTCCTCGACGTGCG
CTCCGACCGCGACCCCAGGTCAGGCGGGACTACCCGCTGA
```

Fig. 8.5 Example of FASTA format of a DNA sequence. It consists of a description line that starts with “>” symbol followed by the identifier of the sequence, and lines of sequences data

8.8 DNA Sequence Alignment

Sequence alignment is an algorithm to arrange two sequences in the highest similarity way in order to locate the differences between them. When the analysis involves more than two sequences, it is called multiple sequence alignment. Sequence alignment can be subdivided into local (Sect. 8.8.1) and global (Sect. 8.8.2) ones according to the way of comparison. BLAST and Clustal are analyzing tools implemented with local and global alignment algorithm, respectively (BLAST also provides a global alignment tool and please refer to Sect. 8.8.2).

8.8.1 Blast

BLAST (http://blast.ncbi.nlm.nih.gov) is a sequence comparison tool in NCBI, which lets user to match a query sequence with a database of sequences. In this context, it adopts local alignment algorithm by dividing the whole query sequence into shorter fragments to calculate the degree of similarity between the query and the matched. NCBI offers three categories of BLAST to suit different searching requirements: BLAST assembled genome, basic BLAST and specialized BLAST. Among them, Nucleotide BLAST in basic BLAST is often used for molecular authentication. It is worth mentioning that user needs to adopt one of the three databases [“Human genomic + transcript,” “Mouse genomic + transcript,” and “Others (nr etc.)”]. If wrong databases are chosen, BLAST may give a false negative result. As a thumb of rule, “Others (nr etc.)” database should be selected [unless the medicinal material is derived from human or mouse, such as Hominis Placenta (*Ziheche*)].

User can either paste the sequence into the text field of BLAST page or upload a FASTA file. Upon completion, BLAST will show a search result page consisting of four parts: (a) the information of query sequence and BLAST search criteria specified by the user (Fig. 8.6a); (b) a graphic summary showing alignments

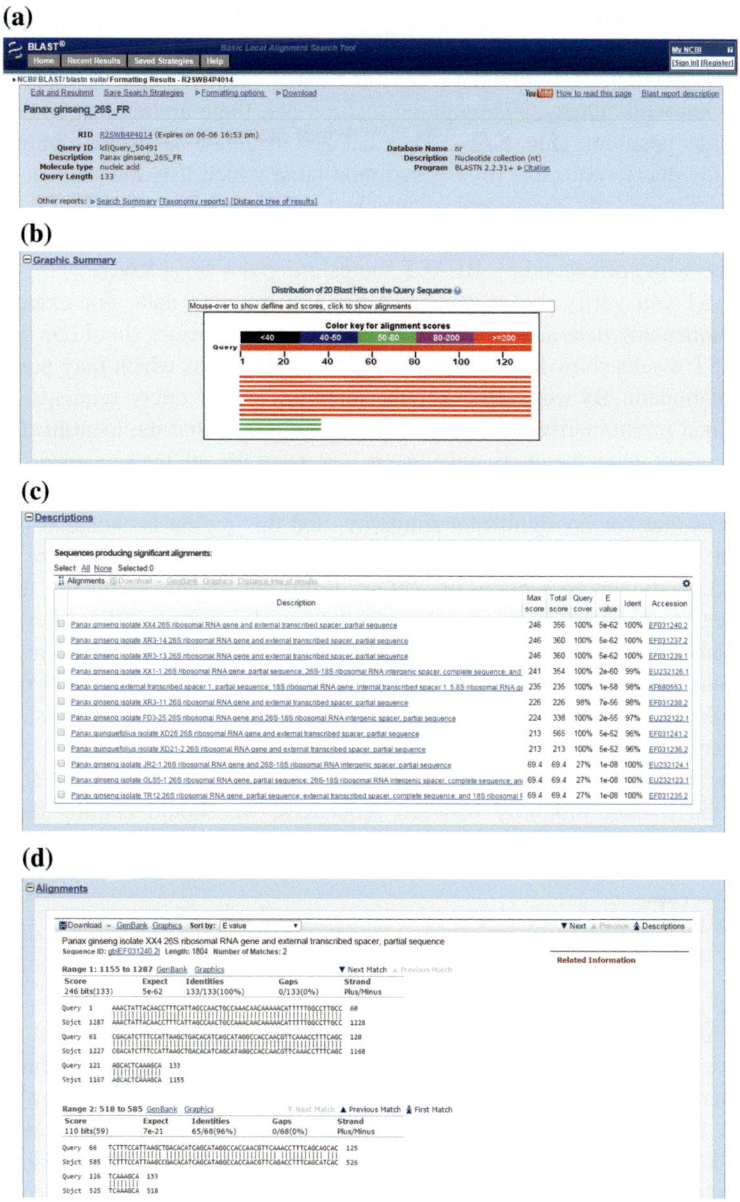

Fig. 8.6 Sequence matching result page of BLAST. After performing a BLAST search on NCBI, it will show a BLAST hits page consisting of four parts. **a** The uppermost part displays the specified criteria, the properties of query sequence and the chosen database. **b** The second part is the graphic summary. The *red bar* marked with "Query" represents the query sequence, and subsequent *bars* are matched database sequences. The *colors* indicates the alignment score within the particular region between the query and matched sequences. **c** In the third part, there is a summary table listing the sequence identifiers, descriptions, and scores of BLAST hits. **d** In the last part, sequence alignment between the query and the matched sequences is given

between query and database sequences. Five color keys (black, blue, green, pink, and red) denote the score ranges of alignment: the black key is the lowest while the red one is the highest. Below these keys, the query sequence is represented as a red bar labeled with "Query." Throughout this red bar, there are numbers indicate the nucleotide positions (Fig. 8.6b). The matched database sequences immediately follow the query sequence; (c) a description table which lists the sequence identifier, description, and the scores of matched database sequences (Fig. 8.6c). The table can be sort by preferred criteria; (d) the alignment between query and database sequence with corresponding BLAST scores are given (Fig. 8.6d).

BLAST can verify the reliability of the experimental data. For example, the DNA sequencing data obtained from a plant or animal species should be discarded if BLAST results show high similarity with fungal species which may possibly be the contaminant. By using BLAST, the identities of the query sequences can be determined preliminarily. However, it must be stressed that the identification may not be correct when the query coverage is low, even though the sequence similarity is shown as 100 %. As a local alignment program, BLAST discards the region of sequences that has no significant similarity, and this region is excluded from calculation. As an extreme example, suppose species A and species B are the two matched candidates to a query of 200 bp. From the graphic summary, the entire sequence of species A is red in color and the length is equal to the query. On the other hand, only the first 100 nucleotides of species B are red, while the rest has no shared similarity to query and thus are blank. In spite of this, BLAST will show that the similarities of two species are 100 % to the query. Under the circumstance, we should conclude that the query sequence is identical to species A but not species B, even the first 100 nucleotides of species B is identical to the query. To accurately reflect the overall similarity between sequences, we should employ the global alignment, which is the topic of the next section.

8.8.2 Clustal

Global alignment is a way of arranging every nucleotide or amino acid in every sequence from beginning to end to identify regions of similarity. Clustal is a computer program developed by Higgins and Sharp [30], which allows global multiple alignment of nucleotide or protein sequences. By uploading the sequences in FASTA format to Clustal, it produces the alignment together with the similarities and phylogenetic tree. Some software packages such as BioEdit [28] incorporates Clustal as a built-in function. BLAST also provides a global alignment tool called Needleman-Wunsch Global Align Nucleotide Sequences.

For sequences with high homology, similar in length, or belong to protein-coding gene (such as *rbcL*), the global alignment result is generally reliable. However, the alignment result needs to be adjusted manually for sequences with low homology, varying amplicon sizes, or from intergenic region (such as ITS or chloroplast intergenic *trnH-psbA* spacer). Like other intergenic spacer regions, the two ends of *trnH-psbA* region are protein-coding genes which are rather conserved. On the other hand, as there is no evolutionary pressure in the intergenic spacer, mutations such as insertion/deletion frequently occur, which result in varying length among species. In fact, our group has found that the length of *trnH-psbA* can range from 233 to 663 bp among herbal species used for 'cooling' beverage (Liangcha) in China [31]. One important rule is that the conserved regions must be aligned properly. Basically, Clustal automatically add gaps into the shorter sequences. Nonetheless, if the intergenic spacers are too varied or the two conserved regions are too far apart, Clustal may not be able to recognize the two conserved ends. Consequently, the conserved region (protein-coding gene) of one species is aligned with the intergenic spacer of another species. Changing the gap penalty may improve the quality of alignment, or the resultant alignment can be adjusted manually.

8.9 Bioinformatics Analysis of DNA Sequences

Sequences similarity (Sect. 8.9.1) and genetic distance (Sect. 8.9.2) are frequently used for calculating the differences between sample and standard sequences.

8.9.1 Sequence Similarity Calculation

The sequence similarity between two sequences is calculated as:

(Identical bases between sequences/total length of sequence) $\times$ 100 % [32]

The online Clustal program can generate a list of similarity for each pair of sequences, nevertheless, it is difficult to calculate values for more than two sequences, such as the intraspecific variation among couples of collected samples. Software package BioEdit [28] can generate sequence similarity matrix. By exporting as CSV format, the matrix can be analyzed in Microsoft Excel.

8.9.2 Genetic Distance Calculation

The second approach is by calculating genetic distance between sample and the reference sequences. For molecular authentication purpose, uncorrected p-distance and Kimura 2-parameter (K2P) model are often employed [33–36]. Phylogenetic tree can be constructed to determine the evolutionary position of the samples within the taxon. Molecular Evolutionary Genetics Analysis (MEGA, http://www.megasoftware.net) is a free phylogenetic software with graphical user interface [37].

For DNA barcoding, species identification is reliable if there is a difference between maximum intraspecific and minimum interspecific distance, and this difference is called DNA barcoding gap. It is recommended that the DNA sequence of identified sample should be compared with its closely related species and adulterants using global alignment algorithm (Sect. 8.8.2). The intraspecific and interspecific distances are then calculated using software. If, unfortunately, there is no DNA barcoding gap, other DNA loci should be employed.

8.10 DNA Fingerprinting

DNA fingerprinting is an approach to identify variable nucleotide sequences in the organism. Unlike DNA barcoding, no sequencing step is involved. The resultant patterns are resolved and visualized using gel or capillary electrophoresis. The identification is made possible by recognizing the unique DNA patterns of the species.

8.10.1 Whole Genome Approach

DNA fingerprinting techniques that assess the whole genome, such as Rapid Amplification Polymorphic DNA (RAPD) [38], Amplified Fragment Length Polymorphism (AFLP) [39], are prone to the quantity and quality of DNA template. The DNA degradation in medicinal materials may result in producing inconsistent profiles. On the other hand, as these techniques compare the entire genome, the resolving power may sometimes higher than that only targeting on a specific DNA region (Sect. 8.10.2). GelQuest (http://www.sequentix.de/gelquest/index.php) and GeneMarker (http://www.softgenetics.com/GeneMarker.html) are software packages which assist in analyzing raw data generated from DNA fingerprinting techniques. They accept various data formats, such as gel image and signals produced from capillary electrophoresis. The program determines the sizes of each DNA band and performs cluster analysis using UPGMA and Neighbor-joining algorithms.

8.10.2 Specific Region Approach

In contrast to RAPD and AFLP, Sequence-Characterized Amplification Region (SCAR, Sect. 8.10.2.1), and PCR-Restriction Fragment Length Polymorphism (PCR-RFLP, Sect. 8.10.2.2) only assess a specific region of genome, and they are, in terms of reproducibility, less sensitive to the deterioration of the DNA template.

8.10.2.1 SCAR

SCAR uses species-specific primers to conduct rapid screening for the target species. Species differentiation can be achieved by the amplification of the polymorphic or varying size fragments. Primers should be experimentally validated for the optimal annealing temperature, occurrence of nonspecific amplification and primer dimers formation. Four factors should be considered to get specific and efficient primers: (a) the bases provide the specificity should be located at the 3′ end of the primer; (b) for sample that is dried, stored for long time or highly processed, the employed DNA region should be kept to a minimum length of size while with sufficient differentiation power; (c) check for the unexpected binding of the primers to other species by using BLAST; (d) follow general primer design guidelines such as those in reference [40], especially avoid the formation of self- or heterodimers. Primer 3 (http://bioinfo.ut.ee/primer3) [41, 42] and OligoAnalyzer (http://sg.idtdna.com/calc/analyzer) are online primer design programs that assess the feasibility of designs according to the properties like melting temperate (Tm), GC content, ΔG of hairpin, self- and heterodimers.

8.10.2.2 PCR-RFLP

PCR-RFLP amplifies a specific region of the genome using universal primers followed by digestion with restriction enzymes. The fingerprinting profiles are determined by the presence or absence of restriction sites on the region. NEBCutter (http://nc2.neb.com/NEBcutter2) analyzes and finds available restriction sites. By comparing the restriction maps of different species, user can choose an appropriate restriction enzyme for the test.

8.11 Concluding Remarks

This chapter describes the application of bioinformatics in molecular authentication of Chinese medicinal materials, introduces the databases and analytical tools, and provides guidelines for obtaining high-quality DNA from herbal materials, and for operating various software programs and designing PCR primers. For molecular authentication of Chinese medicinal materials, a reliable database as reference for sequence comparison is of paramount important. At present, many sequence data disposed to the public database have not been validated. Therefore, it is essential to take caution when using these sequences. With the advancement of DNA analyzing techniques and high-throughput screening methods such as deep sequencing [43] and DNA microarray [44, 45] many DNA sequences can be determined simultaneously. These will be useful for analyzing multicomponent medicinal products and broaden the use of DNA technology in authentication and quality control of Chinese medicinal materials.

References

1. Luscombe NM, Greenbaum D, Gerstein M. What is bioinformatics? A proposed definition and overview of the field. Methods Inf Med. 2001;40(4):346–58.
2. Hogeweg P, Hesper B. Interactive instruction on population interactions. Comput Biol Med. 1978;8(4):319–27.
3. Hogeweg P. The roots of bioinformatics in theoretical biology. PLoS Comput Biol. 2011;7(3): e1002021.
4. Watson JD, Crick FH. Molecular structure of nucleic acids: a structure for deoxyribose nucleic acid. Nature. 1953;171(4356):737–8.
5. Fleischmann RD, Adams MD, White O, Clayton RA, Kirkness EF, Kerlavage AR, Bult CJ, Tomb JF, Dougherty BA, Merrick JM, et al. Whole-genome random sequencing and assembly of *Haemophilus influenzae* Rd. Science. 1995;269(5223):496–512.
6. State Pharmacopoeia Commission. Pharmacopoeia of the People's Republic of China: part 1. Beijing: China Medical Science Press; 2010.
7. Editorial Team. National Center for Biotechnology Information. Published on the Internet http://www.ncbi.nlm.nih.gov. Accessed 1 June 2015.
8. Lou SK, Wong KL, Li M, But PP, Tsui SK, Shaw PC. An integrated web medicinal materials DNA database: MMDBD (Medicinal Materials DNA Barcode Database). BMC Genom. 2010;11:402.
9. Hebert PD, Cywinska A, Ball SL, deWaard JR. Biological identifications through DNA barcodes. Proceedings Biological Sciences/The Royal Society. 2003;270(1512):313–21.
10. Zhang GJ. Methodology for Chinese medicine authentication research. Beijing: People's Medical Publishing House; 2010.
11. Swango KL, Timken MD, Chong MD, Buoncristiani MR. A quantitative PCR assay for the assessment of DNA degradation in forensic samples. Forensic Sci Int. 2006;158(1):14–26.
12. Radstrom P, Knutsson R, Wolffs P, Lovenklev M, Lofstrom C. Pre-PCR processing: strategies to generate PCR-compatible samples. Mol Biotechnol. 2004;26(2):133–46.
13. Dellaporta S, Wood J, Hicks J. A plant DNA minipreparation: version II. Plant Mol Biol Rep. 1983;1(4):19–21.
14. Kang H, Cho Y, Yoon U, Eun M. A rapid DNA extraction method for RFLP and PCR analysis from a single dry seed. Plant Mol Biol Rep. 1998;16(1):90.
15. Draper J, Scott R. The isolation of plant nucleic acids. In: Draper J, Scott R, Armitage P, Walden R, editors. Plant genetic transformation and gene expression. A Laboratory Manual, Blackwell, London; 1988. p. 199–236.
16. Lindahl BD, Nilsson RH, Tedersoo L, Abarenkov K, Carlsen T, Kjoller R, Koljalg U, Pennanen T, Rosendahl S, Stenlid J, Kauserud H. Fungal community analysis by high-throughput sequencing of amplified markers—a user's guide. New Phytol. 2013;199 (1):288–99.
17. Sambrook J, Russell DW. Molecular cloning: A laboratory manual. 3rd ed. New York: Cold Spring Harbor Laboratory Press; 2001.
18. CBOL Plant Working Group. A DNA barcode for land plants. Proc Natl Acad Sci USA. 2009;106(31):12794–7.
19. Schoch CL, Seifert KA, Huhndorf S, Robert V, Spouge JL, Levesque CA, Chen W. Nuclear ribosomal internal transcribed spacer (ITS) region as a universal DNA barcode marker for Fungi. Proc Natl Acad Sci USA. 2012;109(16):6241–6.
20. Ye HG, Zou B. Chinese medicinal plants. Beijing: Chemical Industry Press; 2014.
21. eFloras. Flora of China. Missouri Botanical Garden, St. Louis, MO & Harvard University Herbaria, Cambridge, MA. Published on the Internet http://www.efloras.org (2008). Accessed 1 June 2015.

22. European Bioinformatics Institute. EMBL Nucleotide Sequence Database. Published on the Internet http://www.embl.org. Accessed 1 June 2015.
23. Center for Information Biology and DNA Data Bank of Japan. DNA Data Bank of Japan. Published on the Internet http://www.ddbj.nig.ac.jp. Accessed 1 June 2015.
24. Ratnasingham S, Hebert PD. Bold: the barcode of life data system. Mol Ecol Notes. 2007;7(3):355–64. http://www.barcodinglife.org.
25. Altschul SF, Madden TL, Schaffer AA, Zhang J, Zhang Z, Miller W, Lipman DJ. Gapped BLAST and PSI-BLAST: a new generation of protein database search programs. Nucleic Acids Res. 1997;25(17):3389–402.
26. Thompson JD, Higgins DG, Gibson TJ. CLUSTAL W: improving the sensitivity of progressive multiple sequence alignment through sequence weighting, position-specific gap penalties and weight matrix choice. Nucleic Acids Res. 1994;22(22):4673–80.
27. Edgar RC. MUSCLE: multiple sequence alignment with high accuracy and high throughput. Nucleic Acids Res. 2004;32(5):1792–7.
28. Hall TA. BioEdit: a user-friendly biological sequence alignment editor and analysis program for Windows 95/98/NT. Nucleic Acids Symp Ser. 1999;45:95–8.
29. W3C. XML technology. Published on the Internet http://www.w3.org/standards/xml. Accessed 1 June 2015.
30. Higgins DG, Sharp PM. CLUSTAL: a package for performing multiple sequence alignment on a microcomputer. Gene. 1988;73(1):237–44.
31. Li M, Wong K, Chan W, Li J, But P-H, Cao H, Shaw P-C. Establishment of DNA barcodes for the identification of the botanical sources of the Chinese 'cooling' beverage. Food Control. 2012;25(2):758–66.
32. European Bioinformatics Institute. ClustalW help file. Published on the Internet http://www.ebi.ac.uk/Tools/msa/clustalw2/help/faq.html#21. Accessed 1 June 2015.
33. Ha WY, Reid DG, Kam WL, Lau YY, Sham WC, Tam SY, Sin DW, Mok CS. Genetic differentiation between fake abalone and genuine Haliotis species using the forensically informative nucleotide sequencing (FINS) method. J Agric Food Chem. 2011;59(10):5195–203. doi:10.1021/jf104892n.
34. Kress WJ, Wurdack KJ, Zimmer EA, Weigt LA, Janzen DH. Use of DNA barcodes to identify flowering plants. Proc Natl Acad Sci USA. 2005;102(23):8369–74.
35. Guo X, Wang X, Su W, Zhang G, Zhou R. DNA barcodes for discriminating the medicinal plant *Scutellaria baicalensis* (Lamiaceae) and its adulterants. Biol Pharm Bull. 2011;34(8):1198–203.
36. Liu Z, Chen KL, Luo K, Pan HL, Chen SL. DNA barcoding in medicinal plants Caprifoliaceae. China J Chin Materia Medica. 2010;35(19):3527.
37. Tamura K, Peterson D, Peterson N, Stecher G, Nei M, Kumar S. MEGA5: molecular evolutionary genetics analysis using maximum likelihood, evolutionary distance, and maximum parsimony methods. Mol Biol Evol. 2011;28(10):2731–9.
38. Williams JG, Kubelik AR, Livak KJ, Rafalski JA, Tingey SV. DNA polymorphisms amplified by arbitrary primers are useful as genetic markers. Nucleic Acids Res. 1990;18(22):6531–5.
39. Vos P, Hogers R, Bleeker M, Reijans M, van de Lee T, Hornes M, Frijters A, Pot J, Peleman J, Kuiper M, et al. AFLP: a new technique for DNA fingerprinting. Nucleic Acids Res. 1995;23(21):4407–14.
40. PREMIER Biosoft. PCR primer design guidelines. Published on the Internet http://www.premierbiosoft.com/tech_notes/PCR_Primer_Design.html. Accessed 1 June 2015.
41. Untergasser A, Cutcutache I, Koressaar T, Ye J, Faircloth BC, Remm M, Rozen SG. Primer3–new capabilities and interfaces. Nucleic Acids Res. 2012;40(15):e115.
42. Koressaar T, Remm M. Enhancements and modifications of primer design program Primer3. Bioinformatics. 2007;23(10):1289–91.

43. Coghlan ML, Haile J, Houston J, Murray DC, White NE, Moolhuijzen P, Bellgard MI, Bunce M. Deep sequencing of plant and animal DNA contained within traditional Chinese medicines reveals legality issues and health safety concerns. PLoS Genet. 2012;8(4): e1002657.
44. Cheung VG, Morley M, Aguilar F, Massimi A, Kucherlapati R, Childs G. Making and reading microarrays. Nat Genet. 1999;21(1 Suppl):15–9.
45. Duggan DJ, Bittner M, Chen Y, Meltzer P, Trent JM. Expression profiling using cDNA microarrays. Nat Genet. 1999;21(1 Suppl):10–4.

Chapter 9
Proteomic Response Fingerprinting (ProReF) for Rapid Identification of Protein Targets for Chinese Medicine

Yuanyuan Cheng, Jia Zhao and Jianhui Rong

Abstract Chinese medicine (CM) has been used as the clinical therapies for thousands of years in China. The chemical complexity of Chinese medicines makes it difficult to dissect the molecular mechanisms by single-target based approaches. Proteomics is a recently emerged powerful technology for simultaneous detection of multiple protein targets in the cells and tissues. Proteomic response fingerprinting (ProReF) approach uses 2-D SDS-PAGE and MALDI-TOF mass spectrometry to examine the effects of Chinese medicines on the expression levels of various cellular proteins in the cell cultures or animal organs/tissues. In practical, following the treatments with/without Chinese medicines, the protein lysates are analyzed by two-dimensional gel electrophoresis (2-DE). Based on the change of signal intensity, specific protein spots are selected and subsequently identified by mass spectrometry (MS) techniques. The selected proteins are systematically identified and quantitated as the cellular responses to CM. Proteomic information is important for the investigation of target proteins and relevant signaling pathways, thereby facilitating the understanding on the mechanism of action of CM. Here we reviewed the application of proteomics to discover the molecular mechanisms underlying the pharmacological activities of CM formula. We discussed the basic principles and useful protocols for proteomic analyses. We provided detailed procedures for sample preparation (control and CM-treated group), 2-D gel electrophoresis, image comparison, spot excision, trypsin digestion, mass spectrometry identification, and bioinformatics analysis. We also discussed the cellular and molecular approaches for characterizing the regulation of protein expression by active compounds. We anticipate that the readers will easily adapt these procedures for their discoveries of the target proteins for the active CM compounds of interest.

Y. Cheng · J. Zhao · J. Rong (✉)
School of Chinese Medicine, University of Hong Kong, Hong Kong, China
e-mail: jrong@hku.hk

Y. Cheng
e-mail: u3003162@hku.hk

J. Zhao
e-mail: zhaojia7@hku.hk

S. Leung and H. Hu (eds.), *Evidence-based Research Methods for Chinese Medicine*, DOI 10.1007/978-981-10-2290-6_9

Keywords Proteomic response fingerprinting · Chinese medicine · Two-dimensional gel electrophoresis · Mass spectrometry identification

9.1 Introduction

Traditional Chinese medicine (CM) has been widely used to treat various diseases for several thousands of years in China. Over the time, CM has gradually evolved as a unique clinical medical theory involving the diagnosis, treatment, and prevention of diseases. However, CM has not been globally accepted as the standard clinical therapy due largely to the elusive pharmacology of most CM formulas [2]. In practice, a Chinese medicine practitioner often uses the raw medicinal materials, which may not be incompatible with the criteria of Western medicine. In the complex formula, each individual herb may have multiple active components. Such chemical complexity largely hinders the study of the mechanism of action of CM. Fortunately, several different types of modern omics technologies have recently emerged to bridge the gap between CM pharmacology and modern pharmacology.

Omics including genomics, epigenomics, proteomics, and metabolomics are modern systems biology technologies for deciphering the complex interactions between different biological components. Proteomics is a powerful technology to investigate the expression, post-translational modifications, and the interaction networks of a large number of proteins under different biological conditions [14]. Proteomic techniques hold enormous potential to identify drug-targeted proteins and elucidate the mechanism of action of drugs. With the integration of different proteomic analytical techniques including two-dimensional gel electrophoresis (2-DE) and tandem mass spectrometry (MS) technologies, proteomics provides a systematically quantitative and qualitative map of evidence to identify the drug-altered proteins and further uncover the relevant signaling pathways. Post-translational modifications occur with disease progression or drug treatment, and subsequently influence protein functions and the protein–protein interactions [11, 23]. Thus, proteomics is a robust and versatile technology for the investigation of the molecular mechanisms underlying the pharmacological actions of CM. Importantly, the altered patterns of protein expressions constitute the fingerprints of the cellular responses to CM treatment. Such fingerprints represent the global, quantitative, and objective information for the pharmacological activities of CM drugs.

In the present chapter, we reviewed the recent applications of proteomics in the characterization of the pharmacological activities of CM and the underlying molecular mechanisms, discussed the basic principles and provided several useful protocols for general proteomic analysis. Recently, proteomic analysis could use the proteins after labeling with the methods such as stable isotope labeling, mass tag labeling, and fluorescent labeling [15]. Both isotope labeling and mass tag labeling introduce combinatorial heavy isotopologues of C, N, H, and O into proteins via chemical derivation for the measurement and differentiation by mass spectrometry [18].

In contrast, fluorescent labeling is detected by fluorescence imagers [7]. All of these labeling methods are used to monitor biological processes, enhance the detection sensitivity, and locate the site of protein modification. Based on our previous applications of proteomics, we introduced the proteomic response fingerprinting (ProReF) approach involving sample preparation, 2-D gel electrophoresis, comparison, spot excision, trypsin digestion, mass spectrometric identification, and bioinformatic data mining. We also introduced some cellular and molecular approaches for characterizing the modulation of protein expression by CM active components.

9.2 Increasing Use of Proteomics in the Study of Complex CM Drugs

Proteomics has been previously applied to study the mechanisms of action of CM drugs against different diseases such as cancer, inflammation, neurological diseases, and diabetes as summarized in Table 9.1. First, a large number of CM drugs were recently reported to have anticancer effects. However, the specific anticancer mechanisms for these CM drugs have not been fully investigated. We recently compared the proteomic profiles of human HepG2 cells with or without the treatment with astragaloside IV, the major saponin from *Radix Astragali* [16]. Our results demonstrated that astragaloside IV inhibited the colonogenic survival and anchorage-independent growth in HepG2 cells via downregulating the expression of oncogenes such as Vav3.1. As another example, curcumin, which is isolated from *Curcuma longa* L., is well known for its potential of cancer chemoprevention. By employing proteomic approach, Fang and his colleagues identified 12 proteins including acetylhydrolase IB subunit beta, eIF3i, ERP29, SF2/ASF, TDP-43, 3-PGDH, platelet-activating factor in human breast MCF-7 cells after exposure to cucurmin [5]. These proteins were annotated to specific biological processes such as DNA transcription, mRNA splicing, protein degradation, protein folding, protein synthesis, protein translocation, and cell motility. Presumably, curcumin exhibited anticancer activities via regulating most of 12 specific proteins. Similarly, Liu et al. [10] also employed the proteomics approach to demonstrate that triptolide from *Tripterygium wilfordii* inhibited colon cancer growth via altering the expression of 14-3-3 epsilon. Others have already demonstrated that 14-3-3 epsilon is an important regulatory protein in cell cycle and apoptosis [13]. It was found that *Garcinia oblongifolia* attenuated the proliferation of hepatoma cellular carcinoma (HCC) cells [10]. By systematic proteomic analysis, Fu et al. [6] discovered that 1,3,6,7-tetrahydroxyxanthone (TTA), one of the active compounds from *G. oblongifolia*, inhibited cell growth by increasing the expression of p16 and 14-3-3σ.

Second, inflammation is one of the most common target diseases for various CM drugs. Following proteomic analysis with 2-DE and matrix-assisted laser desorption/ionization time of flight mass spectrometry (MALDI-TOF-MS), Sun et al. [21] found that *Salvia miltiorrhiza* polysaccharides suppressed

Table 9.1 The representative proteomics studies of the mechanisms underlying the actions of CM against different disease

CM or active compound	Type of disease	Animal or cell model	Target protein	References
Curcuma longa L. (Curcumin)	Breast cancer	MCF-7 cell line	TDP-43,SF2/ASF, eIF3i, 3-PGDH and ERP29	[5]
Tripterygium wilfordii Hook. f. (Triptolide)	Colon cancer	SW480 cell line	14-3-3ξ	[10]
Garcinia oblongifolia Champ. et Benth. (1,3,6,7-tetrahydroxyxanthone)	Hepatocellular carcinoma	HepG2 cell line	P16 and 14-3-3s	[6]
Salvia miltiorrhiza (polysaccharide)	Immunological liver injury	LPS-induced mice	PRDX6	[21]
Xiao-Qing-Long-Tang	Allergic airway inflammation	OVA-sensitized allergic airway inflammation model mice	Spectrin α2	[12]
Acanthopanax senticosus	Neuroinflammation	BV-2 cell line	SOD2, PRDX1	[8]
Tao-Hong-Si-Wu Decoction	Cerebral ischemia-reperfusion injury	PC12 cell line	Nrf2-mediated phage II enzymes	[17]
Alpinia oxyphylla (protocatechuic acid chrysin)	Parkinson's disease	Zebrafish and PC12 cell line	HO-1 and neuolin	[25]
Xiao Yao San	Depression	Rats	PP2A	[27]
Tian-Qi-Jiang-Tang Capsule	Type 2 diabetes mellitus	Alloxan-induced Wistar rats	Transthyretin and haptoglobin	[24]
Zi-Bu-Pi-Yin	Type 2 diabetes mellitus	Streptozotocin (STZ)-induced diabetic SD rats	PDHE1a and DRP-2	[19]

proinflammatory NF-κB activity via upregulating peroxiredoxin 6 (PRDX6) expression in a mouse model of immunological liver injury induced by lipopolysaccharide (LPS). Xiao-Qing-Long-Tang decoction is a famous classical CM formulation for the clinical treatment of allergic bronchial asthma. In the mouse model of ovalbumin-sensitized allergic airway inflammation, Xiao-Qing-Long-Tang attenuated lung inflammation. Nagai et al. [12] demonstrated the critical role of spectrin α2 downregulation in the anti-inflammatory activities of Xiao-Qing-Long-Tang decoction by proteomics analysis. Moreover, Jiang et al. [8] also investigated the anti-neuroinflammatory activities of *Acanthopanax senticosus* extract (ASE) by proteomic analysis. As a result, ASE appeared to significantly affect a total of 17 proteins in mouse microglial cell line BV-2 under LPS-induced nitrosative stress.

Third, enormous effort has been made to dissect the pharmacological potential of CM remedies in the treatment of stroke, Parkinson's diseases, Alzheimer's disease, and major depression. We recently employed proteomics to identify the protein targets for the botanical active compounds such as amygdalin from *Semen Persicae* and puerarin from *Radix puerariae lobatae*. We demonstrated amygdalin exhibited the neuroprotective and neuritogenic activities via upregulating calcium-binding chaperone calreticulin expression [3]. Our results suggest that puerarin may reduce NO-mediated mitochondrial damage in PC12 cells and primary rat midbrain neurons via inducing arginase 2 as an endogenous mechanism [26]. Tao-Hong-Si-Wu decoction (THSWD) is widely used to treat cerebrovascular disease in China. By analyzing 2-D gel electrophoresis-based proteomic profiles, Qi et al. [17] found that THSWD regulated Nrf2-mediated phase II enzymes to protect PC12 cells against the injury induced by oxygen-glucose deprivation-reperfusion (OGD-Rep). Zhang et al. [25] discovered that the combination of protocatechuic acid and chrysin from *Alpinia oxyphylla* significantly suppressed neurotoxin-induced loss of dopaminergic neurons in zebrafish and mice. Further proteomic analysis revealed that protocatechuic acid and chrysin synergistically upregulated nucleolin and heme oxygenase-1 (HO-1) expression as the important neuroprotective mechanism. Xiao Yao San (XYS) is another classical CM formula for the treatment of mood disorders. Zhu et al. [27] suggested that XYS improved depression-like behaviors in rats treated with chronic upredictable mild stress (CUMS) by suppressing the induction of pyrophosphatase (inorganic) 2 (PPA2). PPA2 is a multimeric protein complex involving structural A subunit, targeting B subunits and catalytic C subunit. The hippocampal level of PPA2 was upregulated by CUMS, whereas XYS prevented such increase of PPA2 expression.

Fourth, type 2 diabetes mellitus (T2DM) is characterized by high blood glucose level and insulin resistance. Importantly, CM drugs showed therapeutic potential in the treatment of chronic disease including T2DM. Proteomic analysis revealed that Tian-Qi-Jiang-Tang capsule improved the diabetic symptoms by downregulating haptoglobin and transthyretin expression [24]. Moreover, Shi et al. [19] used a fluorescence-based differential gel electrophoresis method to investigate the effect of Zi-Bu-Pi-Yin recipe on the hippocampus in a rat model of diabetic cognitive decline. Based on the fold of change, nine protein spots were determined by mass spectrometry. It turned out that Zi-Bu-Pi-Yin recipe affected dystrophin related protein 2 (DRP-2), pyruvate dehydrogenase E1 (PDHE1α) and other closely related proteins in the regulation of energy metabolism, cytoskeleton regulation, and oxidative stress.

These studies mainly focused on the differential expression of specific signaling proteins in selective diseases. Proteomic approach has made it possible to identify the target proteins for complex CM drugs. Nevertheless, successful application of proteomic approach to study CM drugs should consider the following issues. First, the selection of disease models (e.g., human, animal cell lines, and animal models) is critical for sample collection. A disease model should be selected according to the CM theory and the literatures. A good model should be well responsive to CM treatment at the protein level, while false positive results should be prevented. Second, the sensitivity of protein detection should be high enough to allow the collection of the maximal protein spots as the cellular response to CM drugs. Thus, the sensitive method should be chosen to stain the proteins in gels. Third, peptide-based identification of the proteins should be against different database, such as NCBInr and SWISS-PROT. Cross-database examination ensures more information and better accuracy in the identification of proteins. Finally, functional annotation of the identified proteins by bioinformatics should adhere to the therapeutic claims of CM drugs. It is well known that CM drugs may likely influence on multiple protein targets and signaling pathways. The identified proteins should be examined by the software platforms (e.g., STRING and KEGG) for the possible networks of protein–protein interactions and different pathways. Currently, National Institute of Health (NIH) of the USA established a network-based information library on the biological alterations in gene expression and other cellular process due to the exposure to perturbing agents (http://www.lincsproject.org/). Careful comparison between CM drugs and the perturbing agents in this database would be helpful to predict the potential mechanisms underlying the actions for CM drugs.

9.3 Experimental Design

Over the past several years, we have applied the proteomic response fingerprinting (ProReF) method (Fig. 9.1) to study the anticancer and neurological mechanisms of three different CM drugs. We have successfully demonstrated that: (1) astragaloside IV inhibited the growth and metastasis of cancer cells via downregulating the expression of oncogene Vav3.1 [16]; (2) amygdalin elicited the neurogenic and neuroprotective activities by regulating the expression of calreticulin and several other proteins [3]; (3) puerarin inhibited 6-OHDA-induced neurotoxicity via inducing arginase 2 expression [26]. The general ProReF procedure was illustrated in Fig. 9.1, which involves sample preparation, 2-D gel electrophoresis, image comparison, spot extraction, trypsin digestion, mass spectrometry identification, and bioinformatics analysis. In this chapter, we intended to demonstrate how

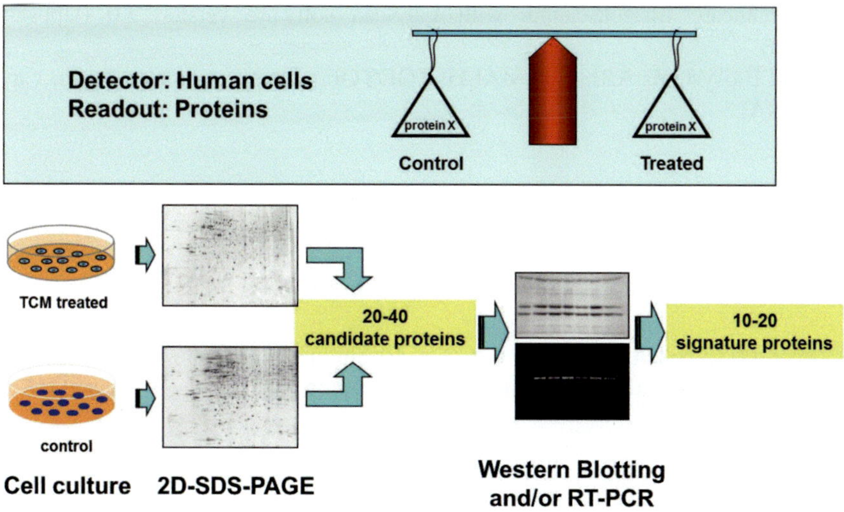

Fig. 9.1 Schematic illustration of proteomic response fingerprinting (ProReF) approach for studying the mechanism of action of CM drugs

ProReF approach was applied to define the mechanism of action of CM drugs, with special emphasis on amygdalin.

9.4 Materials and Methods

9.4.1 Regents

Amygdalin was obtained from Sigma-Aldrich (St. Louis, MO, USA). Antibodies for calreticulin, heat shock protein 90 beta (Hsp90β), 14-3-3ζ/δ, 14-3-3η, glucose-regulated protein 94 (Grp94), and glyceraldehyde 3-phosphate dehydrogenase (GAPDH) were purchased from Cell Signaling Technology (Boston, MA, USA). Antibody against Rab GDP dissociation inhibitor alpha (RabGDIα) was purchased from Santa Cruz Biotechnologies (Santa Cruz, CA, USA). Calreticulin siRNA, control siRNA, and HiPerFect Transfection Reagent were purchased from Qiagen (Hilden, Germany). The neurite outgrowth staining kit was obtained from Invitrogen (Carlsbad, CA, USA).

9.4.2 Instruments

Eppendorf Centrifuge 5417R (Hamburg, Germany)
Bio-Rad Microplate Reader Model 680 (Hercules, CA, USA)
GE Healthcare EttanIPGphor 3 apparatus (Uppsala, Sweden)

GE Healthcare ImagerScanner with LabScan software version 5.0 (Uppsala, Sweden)
Applied Biosystems ABI 4800 MALDI-TOF/TOF mass spectrometer (Foster City, CA, USA).

9.4.3 *Experimental Procedures*

9.4.3.1 Preparation of Samples (Duration 1–4 Days)

1. Seed PC12 cell at the density of 0.3 × 10^5/ml in 10-cm dishes. After overnight incubation, culture the cells in the differentiation medium (1 % HS and 0.5 % FBS) for 24 h.
   - *CRITICAL STEP*: Cell density may affect the outcomes of ProReF studies. The appropriate density of cells should be selected for specific cell lines.
2. Treat the cells with amygdalin (5 μM) in differentiation medium at 37 °C for 3 days, while vehicle was used as control.
   - *CRITICAL STEP*: The drug concentration should be titrated based on the cytotoxicity. The subtoxic concentration should be used in ProReF studies.
3. Wash the cells twice with 1× PBS solution when drug treatment is done.
4. Add 1 ml trypsin to the cell culture, incubate at 37 °C for 5 min, and then harvest the cells by centrifugation at 1000×*g* for 5 min.
5. Wash the cell pellets twice with 10 mM Tris-HCl buffer (pH 7.0) containing 250 mM sucrose.
6. Lyse the cells by incubating the cells in 300 μl lysis buffer containing 40 mM Tris, 65 mM dithiothreitol (DTT), 8 M urea, 2 % ampholine and 4 % CHAPS at 4 °C for 30 min.
7. Centrifuge the mixture at 15,000×*g* for 15 min at 4 °C, collect the supernatant as the cellular proteins for analysis, and measure the protein concentration by the Bradford assay.

9.4.3.2 Two-Dimensional (2-D) Gel Electrophoresis (Duration 28–29 h)

1. Run the 2-D gel electrophoresis according to the manufacturer's instructions from GE Healthcare (Uppsala, Sweden).
2. Perform isoelectric focusing (IEF) in 24-cm Immobiline Drystrips (pH 3.0–10.0) on an EttanIPGphor 3 apparatus from GE Healthcare (Uppsala, Sweden).

Table 9.2 Optimal sample loads onto IPG strip for silver and Coomassie staining

Immobiline		Suitable sample load (μg of protein)	
Size of dry strip (cm)	pH	Silver stain	Coomassie stain
7	3–10	2–6	10–60
11	3–10	4–8	20–120
13	3–10	8–15	40–240
18	3–10	15–30	75–450
24	3–10	20–40	100–600

- *CRITICAL STEP*: The size of IPG strip should be decided based on the experimental needs and sample load. The range of sample load onto the IPG strip is suggested in Table 9.2.

3. Mix 300 μg of the cellular proteins with rehydration solution containing 10 mM DTT, 2 M thiourea, 7 M urea, 0.5 % immobilized-pH-gradient (IPG) buffer (pH 3.0–10.0), and 2 % CHAPS to make up the total volume of 450 μL.

   - *CRITICAL STEP*: The rehydration solution should be freshly prepared. The total sample volume after the addition of rehydration solution should not exceed the holding capacity of the strip.

4. Load the sample-rehydration solution mixture in the strip holders and overlay each IPG strip with DryStrip Cover Fluid to reduce evaporation and urea crystallization.
5. Treat the IPG strips with the following program: 50 V for 24 h, 500 V for 1 h, 1000 V for 1 h, and 8000 V until the current dropped below 25 μAm, over a total of >100,000 V/h.
6. Equilibrate IPG strips with SDS-Equilibration buffer plus dithiotheritol (DTT) for 20 min reduction, and with SDS-Equilibration buffer plus iodoacetamide (IAA) for another 20 min alkylation.
7. Wash the IPG strips with 1× SDS-PAGE running buffer to remove the excessive DTT and IAA.
8. Place the equilibrated IPG strips onto 2-D gels between the two glass plates. The filter papers were loaded with protein markers and subsequently inserted the two sides of the IPG strips.
9. Add 1 mL of agarose sealing mixture over gel strips and use filter paper to cover them completely. Allow the agarose to be solidified within 10–15 min.
10. Run 12.5 % SDS-PAGE gels at 20 W/gel for 4 h on EttanDalt electrophoresis apparatus from GE Healthcare (Uppsala, Sweden).

    - *CRITICAL STEP*: A suitable voltage should be used to run the gel without causing overheating.

9.4.3.3 Protein Imaging and Comparison (Duration 2–4 h)

1. Stain the gels with a standard silver staining kit (Invitrogen, Carlsbad, CA, USA) or Coomassie Brilliant blue R-250 solution (Rio-rad, USA).
2. For silver staining, fix the gels with 10 % acetic acid in 40 % ethanol for 20 min.
3. Wash the gels with 30 % ethanol and water to decant fixative solution.
4. Incubate the gels in Sensitizing solution for 10 min, 30 % ethanol solution for another 10 min, and wash the gels with water for several times.
5. Incubate the gels in silver staining solution for 15 min, and then in developing solution for 8 min.
6. Add the stopper solution to terminate the reaction after the protein spots were fully developed.
7. For Coomassie blue staining, stain the gels in Coomassie Brilliant blue R-250 solution for 2 h or overnight.
8. Destain the gels for 2 h or longer with multiple changes of the destaining solution (10 % acetic acid in 40 % methanol) until the background is less dark.
9. Scan the stained gels on ImagerScanner with LabScan software version 5.0 (GE Healthcare).
10. Analyze the images through background abstraction, spot intensity calibration, spot detection, edition, and matching by using GE Healthcare ImageMaster Platimum software version 5.0.
11. Quantify the signal intensity of each spot by calculating the spot volume after the gel images were normalized.
12. Compare the spots in control and drug-treated maps, and select the protein spots with significant change of density for further identification.

    - *CRITICAL STEP*: Specifically, the spots for upregulated protein were picked from the drug-treated map, whereas the spots for downregulated proteins were picked from the control group.

9.4.3.4 Spots Extraction and Trypsin Digestion (Duration 1–2 h)

1. Cut the spots of interest on an automated spot picker and remove the silver stain by incubating gel pieces with the destaining solution containing 30 mM potassium hexacyanoferrate and 100 mM sodium thiosulfate (1:1, v/v) for 20 min.

    - *CRITICAL STEP*: The destaining solution should be freshly prepared.

2. Wash the gel pieces twice with water, incubate samples in 100 mM ammonium bicarbonate for 5 min and dehydrate with 100 % acetonitrile.
3. Remove the residual solvent by a vacuum centrifuge.

4. Digest the proteins by 20 μg/mL proteomics sequencing grade trypsin (Promega) in the ice-cold 40 mM ammonium bicarbonate buffer including 9 % acetonitrile.
5. Extract the peptides twice with 5 % formic acid and 50 % acetonitrile for 15 min at room temperature and dry the samples in a vacuum centrifuge.

9.4.3.5 Peptide Identification by MALDI-TOF Mass Spectrometry (Duration 4–6 h)

1. Dissolve the peptide residues in 10 μL of 0.1 % formic acid. After mixing with an equal volume of 10 mg/mL α-cyano-4-hydroxycinnamic acid in 0.1 % formic acid in 50 % acetonitrile, the mixtures were spotted onto the MALDI target plates.
2. Perform the MS measurements on an ABI 4800 MALDI-TOF/TOF mass spectrometer from Applied Biosystems (Foster City, CA).
3. Set the MALDI-TOF parameters for peptide mass fingerprint (PMF) as follows: accelerating voltage, 20 kV; grid voltage, 64.5 %; delay, 100 ns; the number of laser shots, 200; and peptide masses range, 900–4000 Da.
4. Switch MS survey scan to MS/MS, and set collision-induced-dissociation (CID) MS/MS parameters as follows: positive mode, 2 kV, 5 monoisotopic precursors, S/N > 200.
5. Use P14R and oxidized insulin chain B from bovine pancreas (Sigma) for external standards and autolytic trypsin fragments as internal standards for mass calibration.

9.4.3.6 Bioinformatics Analysis (Duration 4–6 h)

1. According to the tryptic fragment sizes, search PMF spectrum data in the SWISS-PROT database (http://www.expasy.org/) or the NCBInr database using Mascot program (http://www.matrixscience.com) for protein identification.
2. Set search parameters as follows: Species (Rats); trypsin digestion (≤ 1 missed cleavage); cysteines modified by carbamidomethylation; methionine modified by oxidation; the mass tolerance of 75 ppm; probability scores of >90.

9.4.3.7 Verification and Mechanism Study

1. Treat the cells with amygdalin or other CM drugs at different concentrations.
2. Verify the expression of the candidate proteins by Western blotting.
3. Explore how the drugs regulate the expression of selected protein and discover the potential implications in the treatment of specific disease.

Example results

At the end of drug treatment with amygdalin and vehicle control, the protein lysates were prepared and resolved by 2-D gel electrophoresis. The representative images are shown in Fig. 9.2 [3]. By comparing the intensity of protein spots in the gel image A (amygdalin-treated) and the gel image B (untreated samples), a total of 11 protein spots were found to be significantly altered, in particular, 9 upregulated protein spots and 6 downregulated protein spots. As shown in Fig. 9.2, the amygdalin affected protein spots were indicated by arrows and indexed by numbers. These protein spots were subsequently picked up, fragmented through in-gel digestion and identified by MALDI-TOF-MS analysis. The individual protein spots were identified and annotated using Mascot software (http://www.matrixscience.com) against NCBInr and Swissprot protein databases.

As shown in Table 9.3, the levels of nine proteins expression were increased after amygdalin treatment. These proteins include 14-3-3ζ/δ (NP_037143), 14-3-3η (NP_037184), calreticulin (NP_071794), elongation factor 1-γ (NP_001004223), hepatoma derived growth factor (NP_446159), Hsp90β (NP_001004082), Grp94 (NP_001012197), Rab GDIα (NP_058784), and γ-actin (NP_001120921). On the other hand, the levels of another two proteins were downregulated by amygdalin, such as α-internexin (NP_062001) and phosphoglycerate mutase-2 (NP_059024).

To verify the effects of amygdalin on the expression levels of selected proteins, we further analyzed six representative proteins including 14-3-3ζ/δ, 14-3-3η, calreticulin, Grp94, Hsp90β and Rab GDIα by Western blotting technique. These proteins were selected based on their biological relevance to neuroprotection and neurogenesis. To understand the regulation of calreticulin expression, we treated PC12 cells with amygdalin at the indicated concentrations (e.g., 0, 2.5, 5, and 10 μM). As shown in Fig. 9.3, amygdalin upregulated the calreticulin expression in

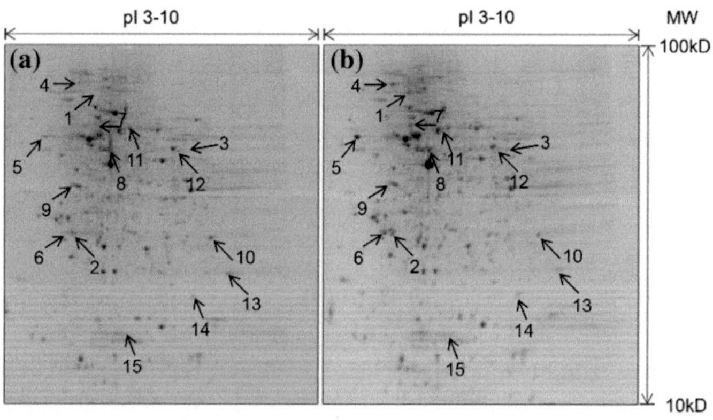

Fig. 9.2 The proteomic maps (2-DE images) of PC12 cells after or before amygdalin treatment. Image **a** represents the proteomic profile from the amygdalin-treated cells, whereas Image **b** represents the proteomic profile from the untreated control cells. The *arrows* pointed to the protein spots selected for MS identification. Reprint with permission from [3]

Table 9.3 MALDI-MS identification of the protein spots that were mostly affected by amygdalin

Spot no.	Protein name	Accession number	MW (KDa)	p*I*	Protein scores	Peptide matches	Fold change
1	Heat shock protein 90β	NP_001004082	83.57	4.97	477	25	+15.78
2	14-3-3η	NP_037184	28.37	4.81	344	12	+4.79
3	Elongation factor-1γ	NP_001004223	50.37	5.42	193	12	+3.70
4	Endoplasmin	NP_001012197	93.00	4.72	636	32	+3.27
5	Calreticulin	NP_071794	48.14	4.33	641	20	+2.68
6	14-3-3ζ/δ	NP_037143	27.92	4.73	574	17	+2.52
7	Rab GDP dissociation inhibitor-α	NP_058784	51.07	5.00	321	17	+2.35
8	Actin, cytoplasmic 2	NP_001120921	42.11	5.31	596	16	+1.79
9	Hepatoma derived growth factor	NP_446159	127.28	5.05	291	9	+1.79
10	Phosphoglycerate mutase 2	NP_059024	28.94	6.67	421	13	−1.74
11	α-Internexin	NP_062001	56.39	5.20	230	15	−4.69

a concentration-dependent manner. The other proteins including 14-3-3ζ, 14-3-3η, Grp94, Hsp90β, and RabGDIα were also validated by Western blotting (Fig. 9.3) [3]. These results were in consistent with the results of 2-DE analyses.

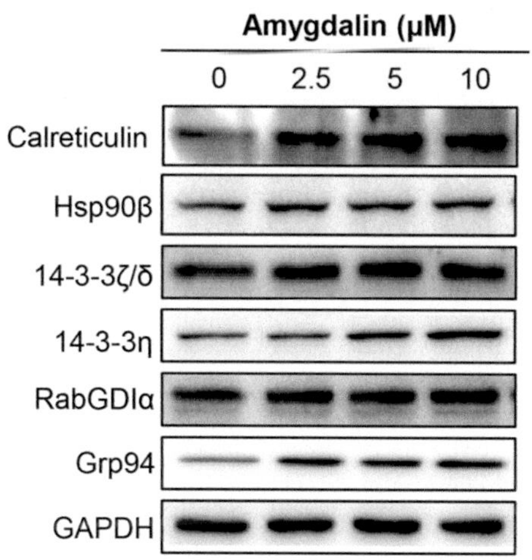

Fig. 9.3 Western blot verification of protein expression in response to amygalin treatment. PC12 cells were treated with amygdalin at the indicated concentrations for 72 h. The cellular proteins were extracted and analyzed by Western blotting. The selected proteins including 14-3-3ζ, 14-3-3η, calreticulin, Grp94, Hsp90β, and rab GDP dissociation inhibitor-α were detected by specific antibodies. Reprint with permission from [3]

9.5 Conclusion

In conclusion, the proteomic approach has been widely used to characterize the biological activities of various CM drugs [4, 9]. Compared with genomics, proteomics provides direct information on the difference in the protein expression in the complex physiological and pathological processes [20]. This review introduced the ProReF approach to promote the process of modernization and globalization of CM drugs. It is undoubtable that ProReF approach will facilitate the integration of proteomics and bioinformatics for the study of protein–drug interactions, protein signaling pathways and disease mechanisms [1]. We believe that better understanding of the networks between the active compounds and the cellular proteins will accelerate the development of evidence-based and mechanism-defined CM drugs [22].

References

1. Altelaar AF, Munoz J, Heck AJ. Next-generation proteomics: towards an integrative view of proteome dynamics. Nat Rev Genet. 2013;14:35–48.
2. Bauer R, Chan K. Special issue: Traditional Chinese medicine. Planta Med. 2010;76:1947.
3. Cheng Y, Yang C, Zhao J, Tse HF, Rong J. Proteomic identification of calcium-binding chaperone calreticulin as a potential mediator for the neuroprotective and neuritogenic activities of fruit-derived glycoside amygdalin. J Nutr Biochem. 2015;26:146–54.
4. Cho WC. Application of proteomics in Chinese medicine research. Am J Chin Med. 2007;35:911–22.
5. Fang HY, Chen SB, Guo DJ, Pan SY, Yu ZL. Proteomic identification of differentially expressed proteins in curcumin-treated MCF-7 cells. Phytomedicine. 2011;18:697–703.
6. Fu WM, Zhang JF, Wang H, Tan HS, Wang WM, Chen SC, Zhu X, Chan TM, Tse CM, Leung KS, Lu G, Xu HX, Kung HF. Apoptosis induced by 1,3,6,7-tetrahydroxyxanthone in Hepatocellular carcinoma and proteomic analysis. Apoptosis. 2012;17:842–51.
7. Griebel A, Obermaier C, Westermeier R, Moche M, Buttner K. Simplification and improvement of protein detection in two-dimensional electrophoresis gels with SERVA HPE lightning red. Arch Physiol Biochem. 2013;119:94–9.
8. Jiang T, Wang Z, Xia ST, Zhao X, Jiang L, Teng L. Quantitative proteomics analysis for effect of *Acanthopanax senticosus* extract on neuroinflammation. Pak J Pharm Sci. 2015;28:313–8.
9. Lao Y, Wang X, Xu N, Zhang H, Xu H. Application of proteomics to determine the mechanism of action of traditional Chinese medicine remedies. J Ethnopharmacol. 2014;155:1–8.
10. Liu Y, Song F, Wu WK, He M, Zhao L, Sun X, Li H, Jiang Y, Yang Y, Peng K. Triptolide inhibits colon cancer cell proliferation and induces cleavage and translocation of 14-3-3 epsilon. Cell Biochem Funct. 2012;30:271–8.
11. Mann M, Jensen ON. Proteomic analysis of post-translational modifications. Nat Biotechnol. 2003;21:255–61.
12. Nagai T, Nakao M, Shimizu Y, Kodera Y, Oh-Ishi M, Maeda T, Yamada H. Proteomic analysis of anti-inflammatory effects of a kampo (Japanese herbal) medicine "Shoseiryuto (Xiao-Qing-Long-Tang)" on airway inflammation in a mouse model. Evid Based Complement Alternat Med. 2011;2011:604196.

13. Nielsen MD, Luo X, Biteau B, Syverson K, Jasper H. 14-3-3 Epsilon antagonizes FoxO to control growth, apoptosis and longevity in Drosophila. Aging Cell. 2008;7:688–99.
14. Oberg AL, Kennedy RB, Li P, Ovsyannikova IG, Poland GA. Systems biology approaches to new vaccine development. Curr Opin Immunol. 2011;23:436–43.
15. Obermaier C, Griebel A, Westermeier R. Principles of protein labeling techniques. Methods Mol Biol. 2015;1295:153–65.
16. Qi H, Wei L, Han Y, Zhang Q, Lau AS, Rong J. Proteomic characterization of the cellular response to chemopreventive triterpenoid astragaloside IV in human hepatocellular carcinoma cell line HepG2. Int J Oncol. 2010;36:725–35.
17. Qi HY, Li L, Yu J, Chen L, Huang YL, Ning L, Jiang Z, Yang N, Xu XY. Proteomic identification of Nrf2-mediated phase II enzymes critical for protection of Tao Hong Si Wu decoction against oxygen glucose deprivation injury in PC12 cells. Evid Based Complement Alternat Med. 2014;2014:945814.
18. Rauniyar N, Yates JR. Isobaric labeling-based relative quantification in shotgun proteomics. J Proteome Res. 2014;13:5293–309.
19. Shi X, Lu XG, Zhan LB, Qi X, Liang LN, Hu SY, Yan Y, Zhao SY, Sui H, Zhang FL. The effects of the Chinese medicine ZiBu PiYin recipe on the hippocampus in a rat model of diabetes-associated cognitive decline: a proteomic analysis. Diabetologia. 2011;54:1888–99.
20. Smith JC, Figeys D. Proteomics technology in systems biology. Mol BioSyst. 2006;2:364–70.
21. Sun XG, Fu XQ, Cai HB, Liu Q, Li CH, Liu YW, Li YJ, Liu ZF, Song YH, Lv ZP. Proteomic analysis of protective effects of polysaccharides from *Salvia miltiorrhiza* against immunological liver injury in mice. Phytother Res. 2011;25:1087–94.
22. Ventura C. CAM and cell fate targeting: molecular and energetic insights into cell growth and differentiation. Evid Based Complement Alternat Med. 2005;2:277–83.
23. Zhang H, Ge Y. Comprehensive analysis of protein modifications by top-down mass spectrometry. Circ Cardiovasc Genet. 2011;4:711.
24. Zhang SX, Sun H, Sun WJ, Jiao GZ, Wang XJ. Proteomic study of serum proteins in a type 2 diabetes mellitus rat model by Chinese traditional medicine Tianqi Jiangtang Capsule administration. J Pharm Biomed Anal. 2010;53:1011–4.
25. Zhang Z, Li G, Szeto SS, Chong C, Quan Q, Huang C, Cui W, Guo B, Wang Y, Han Y, Siu MKW, Lee SM, Chu IK. Examining the neuroprotective effects of protocatechuic acid and chrysin on in vitro and in vivo models of Parkinson's disease. Free Radic Biol Med. 2015;84:331–43.
26. Zhao J, Cheng Y, Yang C, Lau S, Lao L, Shuai B, Cai J, Rong J. Botanical drug puerarin attenuates 6-hydroxydopamine (6-OHDA)-induced neurotoxicity via upregulating mitochondrial enzyme arginase-2. Mol Neurobiol. 2015;53:2200–11.
27. Zhu X, Xia O, Han W, Shao M, Jing L, Fan Q, Liu Y, Diao J, Lv Z, Sun X. Xiao Yao San improves depressive-like behavior in rats through modulation of beta-arrestin 2-mediated pathways in Hippocampus. Evid Based Complement Alternat Med. 2014;2014:902516.

Chapter 10
Chinese Medicines in Neurological Diseases: Pharmacological Perspective

Jia-Hong Lu, Min Li, Ming-Yue Wu and Cui-Zan Cai

Abstract Neurological diseases are a wide range of diseases affecting central and peripheral nervous system. Stroke, Alzheimer's disease (AD), and Parkinson's disease (PD) are the most common and challenging neurological diseases which lack effective treatment. Chinese medicine (CM) is an ancient yet still alive medical system widely used by Asian people for preventing and treating diseases. The symptoms of stroke, AD, and PD have been described in CM books as early as 2000 years ago. The causes as well as the treatment principles for these diseases are also mentioned in the classic CM books. According to CM theory, the diseases are caused by disharmony of *Yin* and *Yang*, thus the treatment strategy is to restore the balance. Throughout the CM history, the etiology and therapy for stroke, AD, and PD have been continuously developed. Currently, Up to 20–40 % of patients with above-mentioned diseases are receiving CM treatment in China, indicating the wide acceptance of CM for the treatment of neurological diseases (Liu in J Am Med Dir Assoc, 2015 [1]; Rajendran et al. in Neurology 57:790–4, 2001 [2]). The widely used formulas for neurological disease treatment include: "Qi Fu Decoction", and "Tongqiao Huoxue Decoction" for Dementia; "Zhengan Xifeng Decoction", "Angong Niuhuang Wan" "Tongqiao Huoxue decoction", "Taohong Siwu Decoction" for Stroke; "Zhengan Xifeng Decoction", "Lingjiao Gouteng Decoction", "Dao Tan Decoction", "Renshen Yangrong Decoction", and "Dihuang Yinzi Decoction" for PD. Numerous studies have reported the efficacy of CM in the clinic treatment of stroke, AD, and PD. However, most of the clinical studies lack the experimental supports from diseases models and the reports were mainly written in

J.-H. Lu (✉) · M.-Y. Wu · C.-Z. Cai
State Key Laboratory of Quality Research in Chinese Medicine, Institute of Chinese Medical Sciences, University of Macau, Macau, China
e-mail: jiahonglu@umac.mo

M.-Y. Wu
e-mail: blackmoon19890103@hotmail.com

C.-Z. Cai
e-mail: caizan617@126.com

M. Li
School of Chinese Medicine, Hong Kong Baptist University, Hong Kong, China
e-mail: limin@hkbu.edu.hk

S. Leung and H. Hu (eds.), *Evidence-based Research Methods for Chinese Medicine*, DOI 10.1007/978-981-10-2290-6_10

Chinese, thus limiting the recognition of CM by worldwide researchers. With the modernization of CM during the past decades, the experimental data of CM-originated materials (formula, herb extract, and single compounds) on the stroke, AD, and PD models are accumulating rapidly, providing important scientific evidence for the clinic use of CM for treating neurological diseases. This chapter introduces the basic theory of CM for treating stroke, AD, and PD, lists the currently used experimental diseases models for the evaluation of pharmacological activity of CM, and summarizes the CM-originated materials with protective effects in these disease models.

Keywords Chinese medicine · Neurological disease · Stroke · Neurodegenerative diseases

10.1 Stroke

Stroke, also known as cerebrovascular accident, is a kind of "brain attack". In America, there are more than 500,000 people attacked by stroke annually, and one American dies from stroke every 4 min [3]. In China, stroke has become the second leading cause of death [4]. Stroke occurs due to interrupted blood supply which results in acute neuronal death in affected regions. Subsequently, stroke symptoms that related to affected brain regions appear. The most common symptoms of stroke are: (1) weakness or numbness of some parts of the body; (2) vision lost; (3) deficiency of talking or comprehensive abilities; (4) sudden severe headache; and (5) balance disability or unstable walking.

Stroke can be classified into two types: ischemic stroke and hemorrhagic stroke. The ischemic stroke is the most common type, occupying about 80 % of all strokes. Ischemic stroke often occurs when cerebral circulation is blocked by clots. Fatty deposits and elevated cholesterol are known to be the major risk factors of clotting. Hemorrhagic stroke is caused by breakage of blood vessels in the brain. High blood pressure and brain aneurysms are risk factors for hemorrhagic stroke.

10.1.1 Stroke Models

10.1.1.1 Animal Models of Stroke

Animal stroke models have long been used to study the pathological mechanism of stroke, and to test the therapeutic interventions. According to the different types and etiologies of stroke, the animal models of stroke can be classified into different types, including ischemic stroke, intracerebral hemorrhage, subarachnoid hemorrhage and cerebral vasospasm, and sinus vein thrombosis. The intracerebral hemorrhage and ischemic stroke are the most widely used ones.

10.1.1.2 Animal Models of Ischemic Stroke

Ischemia animal models are the most commonly used stroke models. There are two mechanistically distinct models of cerebral ischemia: global and focal ischemia. Global ischemia occurs when cerebral blood flow (CBF) is globally interrupted in the brain, while focal ischemia is confined to a specific region of the brain [5]. Models of cerebral ischemia have been established in many species, such as rabbits, dogs, cats, and baboons [6].

To establish global cerebral ischemia model, there are several well-established methods. Neck cuff technique has been used in rats for decades, but there are several complicating factors such as venous congestion and vagal nerve compression, which lead to highly variable ischemic outcomes [5]. Neck cuff inflation plus hypotension technique, a modification of neck cuff technique, has been utilized in monkey and cats. This technique leads to injury in brain stem regions in monkey, but the extent of pathology is different from other primate models [7, 8]. Ventricular fibrillation technique is generally used in large animals, such as dog and pig. It is an excellent and expensive technique, but it would result in whole body ischemia [5]. Four-vessel occlusion (4-VO) model has been well validated and well described. In this model, blood flow in both carotid arteries and vertebral arteries is blocked for a specified time period. It provides a method of reversible forebrain cerebral ischemia, and is produced in awake, freely moving rats [5]. However, the effects of ischemia are variable between rat strains, and the results between laboratories are variable either [5]. The two-vessel (2-VO) model of forebrain ischemia needs bilateral carotid artery occlusion or sometimes along with additional systemic hypotension to produce a reversible forebrain ischemia [5]. In general, the histopathology of this 2-VO model is similar to which occurs in 4-VO model, and the major advantages of the 2-VO model are the simple surgical preparation, readily accomplished reperfusion, and suitability of chronic survival studies [5]. It is worth noting that these models require very careful control of temperature [5].

Focal ischemia models are commonly induced by occlusion of one major cerebral blood vessel such as the middle cerebral artery (MCA) in small or large animals [5]. MCA occlusion (MCAO) occurs at either the proximal or distal part of the vessel. Because the MCAO models are more relevant to human thromboembolic stroke, they have been used extensively. The proximal MCAO can be produced by an intraluminal suture or with a vascular clip and resulting damage to cortex and deep structures [6]. The distal MCAO is usually achieved by placing a vascular clip on a distal vessel or by cautery [6]. In these models, the infarction degrees are usually variable in different rat strains. For instance, Brint et al. [9] found that cortical infarct volume was quite reproducible in SHRs, but not in other strains, when they used MCAO coupled with permanent common carotid artery occlusion. Electrocoagulation and photochemistry are two methods that used to produce ischemia by some investigators. Electrocoagulation technique can reduce cerebral blood flow corresponds closely to the area of neuropathological injury [5]. The photochemical MCAO model that involves the irradiation of some branches of the distal MCA with beams from an argon-dye laser, can achieve consistent infarction in frontoparietal neocortex [5]. However, this photochemical reaction can result in microvascular injury [5]. Blood clot fragments can be injected directly into the carotid artery to form focal ischemia model, but the location of infarction is not consistent [10, 11]. Reperfusion time is another important aspect for these models. Long time of ischemia may appear "no-reflow phenomenon", because of the microvascular occlusion [12]. Moreover, apoptosis in these models is prominent after 30 min MCAO followed by longer reperfusion time [13].

10.1.1.3 Animal Models of Intracerebral Hemorrhage (ICH) Stroke

The most commonly used intracerebral hemorrhage stroke models are intraparenchymal infusion of autologous blood or bacterial collagenase [14]. Blood injection model was designed to mimic the natural events that happen in spontaneous ICH in human, and it is an effective technique to produce an intracerebral hematoma [15]. Collagenase can disrupt the basal lamina of blood vessel, causing blood leak into the surrounding tissue. Considering many patients who undergo continued bleeding or rebleeding, collagenase model may be more appropriate for this hematoma expansion than blood injection model [14]. In addition, collagenase model can easily change the lesion size by varying dose, whereas high blood dose injection may affect lesion shape or cause blood backflow along the injection path [14]. When comparing the progression and extent of injury in these two models, collagenase model results in more severe damage and distant injury in brain than blood injection model [14].

10.1.1.4 Cellular Models of Stroke

Oxygen-glucose deprivation (OGD) has been widely used as an in vitro model for stroke. It mimics the interruption of the supply of oxygen and nutrients to the brain occurring during an ischemic event [16]. Primary neurons culture from different regions of brain can be established from rat or mouse embryos [6]. After deprivation of oxygen and glucose, these cells will display apoptotic and necrotic cell death phenotypes that occur in ischemia [17]. Moreover, cultured brain slices can be also used to study ischemic damage in vitro. For instance, the oxygen and glucose-limited bathing solution would lead to the cell loss in the CA1 region of the brain slice [18].

10.1.2 Stroke from View of Chinese Medicine (CM)

In CM theory, stroke has been called *wind stroke*, which is mainly characterized by sudden collapse, loss of consciousness, facial paralysis, dysphasia, or aphasia [19, 20]. Before the Song dynasty, most CM practitioners believed that the cause of *wind stroke* was related to *external pathogenic wind*. However, after song dynasty, CM practitioners begin to accept the theory that the *wind stroke* is caused by the interrupted *internal wind*, and lead to *Yin* or *Qi* weakness, *liver fire*, *wind-phlegm*, *phlegm-dampness*, or *blood stasis*, following imbalance between *Yin* and *Yang*, deficiency of *liver-Yin* and *Kidney-Yin*, stagnation of *phlegm* and *dampness* [19, 20]. *Wind stroke* can be classified into *Meridian stroke*, *Zang-fu stroke*, and *Sequela*, and the therapeutic approaches would be specifically used for different symptoms [20].

10.1.3 Active Component from CM with Neuroprotective Effects for Stroke

In countries of South and East Asia, CM has been widely used to treat patients with stroke for centuries. Nowadays, the CM are still routinely prescribes for stroke patients, especially in the recovery stage, indicating the therapeutic potentials of CM for stroke. In recent years, a growing number of pharmacological researches have been undertaken to study the effectiveness of CM for stroke [19]. The main mechanisms of therapeutic actions involved in these CM for stroke therapy are: (1) inhibiting inflammatory pathways, such as NF-κB pathway; (2) inhibiting cell apoptosis; (3) alleviating oxidative stress; (4) inhibiting platelet aggregation; (5) attenuating glutamate-induced excitatory toxicity; and (6) increasing the extracellular Gamma Amino Acid Butyric Acid (GABA), and so on.

10.1.3.1 Formula

Unlike some forms of herbalism and western medicine, CM is often used as mixture (formulas) rather than individual drugs to maximize the therapeutic efficacy. It would enhance the effects of individual ingredients, ameliorate adverse side effects, and cover the variation of symptoms [19]. Nowadays, many kinds of formulas treated for stroke have been established (Table 10.1), such as "Hu Xin Dan", "Ren Shen Zai Zao Wan", "An Shen Bu Xin Wan", "Dan Shen Tablets", "Huanglianjiedu Decoction" [21], "Qingxue-dan" [22], "Shenmai san" [23], "Buyang Huanwu Decoction" [24], and so on. Researchers found that these protective abilities may result from their potential roles of ameliorating disturbance in energy metabolism, alleviating oxidative stress and inflammation, and inhibiting apoptosis [21–24].

10.1.3.2 Extract

More than 100 CMs have been used for stroke prevention and therapy by CM practitioners [25]. Some studies have been performed to understand the therapeutic effects of some extracts from CM. A recent research has characterized 58 CMs that are used for the treatment of stroke in vitro [26]. The researchers found that the

Table 10.1 Pharmacological effects of CM on stoke models

Formula/extract/compounds	CM herbs	Model	Drug administration protocol	Pharmacological activity	Mechanism of action	Ref.
70 % ethanol extract of Huang lian jiedu Decoction (黃連解毒湯)	*Coptis chinensis* Franch (黃連), *Scutellaria baicalensis* Georgi (黃芩), *Phellodendron amurense* (黃柏) and *Gardenia jasminoides* J. Ellis (梔子)	MCAO model of SD rats	Suspended in 0.5 % CMC–Na, i.g. at 5.0 g/kg for 10 days	Reduced cerebral infarct area; Ameliorated neurological damage and histopathological abnormality	Ameliorated the disturbance in cellular metabolism, Antioxidative stress, anti-inflammation	[21]
Water extract of Taohong Siwu Decoction (桃紅四物湯)	Radix *Rehmanniae praeparata* (黃芩) Radix *Angelicae Sinensis* (當歸) Rhizoma *Ligustici Chuanxiong* (川芎) Radix *Paeoniae Alba* (白芍) Semen *Prunus* (桃仁) Flos *Carthami Tinctorii* (紅花)	MCAO model of SD rats	p.o. at 0.5, 1.0, and 1.5 g/kg/day for 7 days	Reduced infarct volume and improved neurological function	Activation of PI3K/Akt and the Nrf2 signaling pathway	[115]
80 % ethanol extract of Qingxue-dan (清血丹)	*Scutellaria baicalensis* Georgi (黃芩), *Coptis chinensis* Franch (黃連), *Phellodendron amurense* (黃柏), *Gardenia jasminoides* J. Ellis (梔子) and *Rheum officinale* Baill. (大黃)	Mouse N2a cells Hypoxia (95 % N2/5 % CO_2 for 42 h)	Incubated with cells (50–400 μg/mL) 2 h prior to hypoxia	Decreased the cytotoxicity	Anti-apoptosis	[116]

(continued)

Table 10.1 (continued)

Formula/extract/compounds	CM herbs	Model	Drug administration protocol	Pharmacological activity	Mechanism of action	Ref.
Distilled water extract of Shenmai san (生脈散)	*Panax ginseng* (人蔘), *Ophiopogon japonicus* (麥冬), *Schizandra chinensis* (五味子)	2-VO model of male Wistar rats	Duodenum lumen administration at 5 g/kg 2 h before surgery and 45 min after reperfusion	Improved the oxidative damage during the cerebral ischemia-reperfusion injury	Suppresses the TBARS formation; prevented the loss of glutathione peroxidase activity	[23]
Distilled water extract of Buyang Huanwu Decoction (補陽還五湯)	*Radix angelicae siensis* (白芷), *Radix Paeoniae Rubra* (赤芍), *Rhizoma Chuanxiong* (川芎), *Semen Persicae* (桃仁), *Carthamus tinctorius* L. (紅花) and *Lumbricus* (地龍)	4-VO model of male adult Wistar rats	p.o. at a dose of 6.65 g/kg twice each day for 7 days before ischemia	Less injury in the hippocampal CA1 region; Attenuated the number of TUNEL-positive neurons	Anti-apoptosis	[117]
The supercritical CO_2 and aqueous extracts of FuLing-BaiZhu-DangGui (FBD) (茯苓白朮當歸)	*Wolfiporia extensa* (雲苓), *Atractylodes lancea* rhizome (蒼朮), *Angelica sinensis* (當歸)	2-VO model of male ICR mice	Dissolved in saline, i.g. at 187.5 mg/kg twice per day for 3.5 d prior to surgery	Reduced Evans Blue influx, neuron specific enolase efflux, and brain infarction	Anti-inflammation	[118]
Flavones isolated from methanol extract	*Scutellaria baicalensis* Georgi (黃芩)	4-VO model of male Wistar rats	p.o. at 10 mg/kg after the ischemia induction for 7 days	Inhibited the hippocampal CA1 neuronal damage; Reduced infarct volume	Anti-inflammatory activation of microglia; Antioxidative activity	[27]

(continued)

Table 10.1 (continued)

Formula/extract/compounds	CM herbs	Model	Drug administration protocol	Pharmacological activity	Mechanism of action	Ref.
Flavones isolated from Ethyl acetate extract	*Scutellaria baicalensis* Georgi (黃芩)	MCAO model of male Wistar rats	40–80 mg/kg, (i.p.) at 10 min, 24 h and 36 h after surgery	Protected cerebral hypoxia and reperfusion brain tissues	Inhibites platelet aggregation; Antioxidative activity	[28]
Distilled water extract	Radix *Stephaniae tetrandrae* (防己)	Primary mouse cortical neurons culture (E16)	Half of the medium was replaced with the extract-contained medium every 3–4 days	Attenuated NMDA-induced neurotoxicity	Blockes currents induced by NMDA	[29, 30]
Distilled water extract	Radix *Salviae miltiorrhizae* (丹蔘)	Left coronary artery ligation in male adult Wistar rats	i.p. 15–30 mg/kg 30 min before surgery	Decreased infarct volume	Antioxidative stress	[31]
70 % methanol extract	Ramulus *Uncariae rhynchophylla* (鈎藤)	4-VO model of male adult Wistar rats	100–1000 mg/kg i.p. at 0 and 90 min after reperfusion	Protected hippocampal CA1 neurons damage	Anti-inflammation	[36]
Purified (95 %) total saponins; extracted by steaming at 85 °C	*Panax ginseng* (人蔘)	MCAO model of male Wistar rats or Sprague–Dawley rats	i.p. at 25 mg/kg for 3 days before surgery; i.v. at 45 mg/kg just before surgery	Improved neurological deficits and behavior scores	Neural stem cells activation; antioxidative stress and anti-apoptosis	[33, 34]

(continued)

Table 10.1 (continued)

Formula/extract/compounds	CM herbs	Model	Drug administration protocol	Pharmacological activity	Mechanism of action	Ref.
A standard extract of ginkgo (EGb761)	*Ginkgo biloba* (銀杏)	MCAO model of Sprague-Dawley rats	Before reperfusion, i.v. at 45 mg/kg/day	Increased the ADC value and DCavg value; Improved behavior scores	Enhances phosphorylations of AKT, CREB and the expression of BDNF	[35]
Polysaccharide extract	Radix *Eleutherococcus senticosus* (刺五加)	Modified MCA in male Wistar rats	p.o. at 50–200 mg/kg/day for 15 days before surgery	Improved the symptoms; Reduced the infarct volume and brain water content	Anti-inflammation and antioxidative stress	[36]
85 °C Water extract	*Camellia sinensis (L.)* Kuntze (茶)	MCAO model of male Sprague-Dawley rats	p.o. at 30–300 mg/kg 1 h before surgery	Improved ischemic-induced memory impairment	Antioxidative stress, reduced breakdown of MDA and GSH in brain	[37]
Polysaccharide extract	*Corydalis yanhusuo* (延胡索)	MCAO model of male and female Wistar rats	p.o. at 20–80 mg/kg 60 min before surgery	Improved neurological deficits, reduced the area of cerebral infarct and brain water content	Prolonged clotting time and thrombosis time	[38]
Hydroxysafflor yellow A	*Carthamus tinctorius* L. (紅花)	MCAO model of male Wistar rats	i.v. at 2–8 mg/kg just 15 min after occlusion	Improved neurological deficit and reduced the infarct volume	Antioxidative stress, attenuates the T-AOC	[119]

(continued)

Table 10.1 (continued)

Formula/extract/compounds	CM herbs	Model	Drug administration protocol	Pharmacological activity	Mechanism of action	Ref.
Ginsenoside Rb1	*Panax ginseng* C.A. Mey (人蔘)	Blood clot implanted in the left internal carotid artery in male cynomolgus monkeys	Administered into the cephalic vein of the forearm at 300 μg/kg for 7 days before surgery	Promote neuron survival in the ischemic peri-infarct area	Anti-inflammation and anti-apoptosis	[40]
Ginsenoside Rb1	*Panax ginseng* C.A. Mey (人蔘)	MCAO model of male Sprague-Dawley rats	The intranasal administration at 20 μl solution daily for 1 week before surgery	Alleviated infarction volume and neurological deficit; Inhibits\ed microglia activation	Anti-inflammation	[41]
Bilobalide	*Ginkgo biloba* or *Ginkgo biloba* L. (銀杏)	MCAO model of male Sprague-Dawley rats	i.p. at 10–100 mg/kg, twice 2 and 12 h after the onset of ischemia	Reduced neurological deficit scores and cerebral infarct volume	Anti-inflammation; inhibits apoptosis	[42]
Epigallocatechin gallate	*Camellia sinensis* (L.) Kuntze (茶)	MCAO model of male Sprague-Dawley rats	i.p. at 25 or 50 mg/kg immediately after reperfusion	Reduced the infarction volume, neurological deficit total score	Antioxidative stress	[39]
Puerarin	Radix *Pueraria* (葛根)	MCAO model of male Sprague-Dawley rats	i.p. at 100–400 mg/kg after ischemia and 24 and 48 h after reperfusion	Improved the functional neurological outcome; Inhibited cell damage	Increased the erythropoietin activity	[43]

(continued)

Table 10.1 (continued)

Formula/extract/compounds	CM herbs	Model	Drug administration protocol	Pharmacological activity	Mechanism of action	Ref.
Magnolol	*Magnolia officinalis* Rehder et E.H. Wilson (厚樸)	MCAO model of male Sprague-Dawley rats	i.p. at 25–200 mg/kg pre or after insult	Reduced the infarct volume and improved neurobehavioral outcomes	Restores intracellular Ca^{2+} homeostasis; Attenuated excitatory cytotoxicity	[44]
Protopine	*Papaver somniferum* L. (罌粟), *Corydalis yanhusuo* (延胡索) and *Fumaria officinalis* (球果紫堇)	MCAO model of male Sprague-Dawley rats	i.p. at dose of 0.98–3.92 mg/kg once daily for 3 days before surgery	Reduced the cerebral infarction ratio; Improved the neurological deficit score and histological changes of brain	Increases SOD activity in serum, decreased total calcium and apoptotic cells in brain tissue	[50]
Huperzine A	*Huperzia serrata* (Thunb.) Trevis (蛇足石杉)	MCAO model of male Sprague-Dawley rats	i.p. at dose of 0.1 mg/kg at the onset of occlusion and 6 h later	Restored cerebral blood flow, reduced infarct size and neurological deficit score	Inhibites AChE activity; anti-inflammation	[46]
Schisandrin B	*Schizandra chinensis* (五味子)	MCAO model of male Sprague-Dawley rats	i.p. at 10 or 30 mg/kg 30 min before the surgery or 2 h after the surgery	Reduced the infarct volumes	Anti-inflammation	[47]
Curcumin	*Curcuma longa* L. (薑黃)	MCAO model of male Sprague-Dawley rats	i.p. at a dose of 30–300 mg/kg 30 min after surgery	Reduced infarct volume and cerebral edema	Antioxidative stress; Reduces peroxynitrite formation	[48]

(continued)

Table 10.1 (continued)

Formula/extract/compounds	CM herbs	Model	Drug administration protocol	Pharmacological activity	Mechanism of action	Ref.
Tanshinone II	Radix *Salviae miltiorrhizae* (丹蔘)	MCAO model of male Sprague-Dawley rats	i.p. at 25 mg/kg 10 min after surgery	Diminished infarct volume and brain water content; Improved neurological deficits	Inhibits apoptosis pathway in the ischemic cortex	[49]
Tetrandrine	*Stephania tetrandra* S. Moore	MCAO model of Male Balb/c mice	i.p. at 30 mg/kg immediately or 2 h after surgery	Mitigated cerebral neurological deficits and infarct size; Decreased brain edema	Upregulation of GRP78, DJ-1 and HYOU1	[50]
Gastrodin	*Gastrodia elata* Blume (天麻)	MCAO model of male Sprague-Dawley rats	i.p. at 50 or 100 mg/kg 20 min before surgery	Diminished infarct volume and improved neurological deficits	Decreases the glutamate/GABA ratios	[51]
Theanine	*Camellia sinensis* (L.) Kuntze (茶)	MCAO model of Male ddY mice	i.p. at dose of 1 mg/kg 3 h after occlusion	Reduced the size of cerebral infarct and histological changes of brain	GABAA-receptor activation	[52]
Tetramethylpyrazine	Fermented food natto (納豆)	MCAO model in male Sprague-Dawley rats	i.p. at 10 or 40 mg/kg 60 min before occlusion	Reduced behavioral disturbance; Lowered neuronal loss and brain infarction	Anti-apoptosis; anti-inflammation	[53]
Honokiol	*Magnolia officinalis* Rehder et E.H. Wilson (厚樸)	2-VO model of both male and female Kunming mice	i.p. at 0.7–70 μg/kg immediately after ischemia and 15 min after reperfusion	Reduced brain water contents, decreased the size of cerebral infarct	Anti-inflammation	[54]

protective effects of CM may be attributed to different reasons [27–38]. Extracts of *Radix Scutellariae* baicalensis [27, 28], *Radix Salviae* miltiorrhizae [31], green tea [37] displayed antioxidative activity, *Ramulus Uncariae* [32] can suppress inflammation pathway, and *Acanthopanax senticosus* [36] can both inhibit oxidative stress and inflammatory pathway. *Radix Stephaniae* tetrandrae has been reported to block the currents induced by NMDA [29, 30], and extracts from *ginseng* and *Ginkgo biloba* can enhance the phosphorylation of protein kinase B (Akt), cAMP response element-binding protein (CREB), and the expression of Brain-derived neurotrophic factor (BDNF) in the brains [33, 34]. *Corydalis yanhusuo* can prolong blood clotting time in rats [38]. These pharmacological actions of CM may partially explain its neuroprotective effect for stroke.

10.1.3.3 Single Compounds

In recent years, active compounds from CM have been robustly studied for their pharmacological effect against stroke. Ginsenoside Rb1, Bilobalide, Epigallocatechin gallate [39], Puerarin, Magnolol, Protopine, Huperzine A, Schisandrin B, Curcumin, Tanshinone II, Corynoxeine, Tetrandrine, Gastrodin, Theanine, and Tetramethylpyrazine have been reported to show neuroprotective effects on cerebral ischemia in rodent stroke models [39–54]. These compounds exert their protective activity against ischemia-induced damages by many different mechanisms, such as antioxidative stress, anti-inflammation, inhibiting apoptosis, increasing GABA, activating erythropoietin activity, and so on [39–54].

10.2 Alzheimer's Disease (AD) and Parkinson's Disease (PD)

AD and PD are two most common neurodegenerative disorders which threaten the life quality of the elder [55]. The estimated worldwide prevalence of AD and PD are 5 and 1 % in population over 60 years old. Both AD and PD are associated with depositions of abnormal proteins in the central nervous system (CNS), which resulted in neuronal degeneration and ultimately neuronal death. AD is the major cause of dementia in elder [56], and PD is the leading neurodegenerative movement disorder [57] that destroys the motor function of patients.

10.2.1 Alzheimer's Disease

AD is characterized by progressive impairment of memory and cognitive functions, accompanied by amyloid plaque deposition [58, 59] and neurofibrillary tangles formation [60]. Amyloid plaque is caused by the extracellular accumulation of amyloid beta peptide (Aβ), a 40–42 amino acid peptide generated from series enzymatic cleavage of amyloid precursor protein (APP). Neurofibrillary tangles are formed by aggregation of hyper phosphorylated tau protein. These two events lead to synaptic dysfunction, axon transportation impairment, neuronal dystrophy, inflammation, and finally neuron loss. The most affected regions of AD are hippocampus and cortex. Dementia and psychological symptoms (anxiety, depression, irritability, delusions, and hallucination) are the major clinic features of AD [61]. Along with aging, these symptoms progressively get severe. In other words, age is the principal risk factor for AD [62]. The incidence of the AD doubles every 5 years after 65 years of age, and after 85 years of age the incidence of the disease reach to 30–40 % [63]. Till 2015, there are 46.8 million people suffering from the disease worldwide according to the world Alzheimer report [64].

10.2.1.1 Experiment AD Models

Currently, AD is an incurable disease that lacks effective treatments. Current drug for AD treatment are cholinesterase inhibitors and symptom-relieving agents such as memantine, galantamine, rivastigmine, donepezil, and tacrine. The development of therapeutic intervention to slowdown or reverse the degeneration process is still the biggest challenge for researchers and doctors. Establishment of good model to mimic the pathological features and pathogenesis of AD is a critic step for drug discovery. Many animal models have been developed, including senescence-accelerated mouse model, ischemia-induced model, neurotransmitter-based pharmacological models, AD toxin injection models, and transgenic models. Among these models, transgenic animal model is believed to be the most relevant to AD pathogenesis. The first transgenic animal model was established by Dora Games and his colleagues in 1995. They used platelet-derived growth factor (PDGf)-β promoter to drive human APP expression. The mice express high levels of APP in the brain and develop pathological hallmarks of AD, including Aβ deposition and loss of neurons [65]. The Transgenic mice overexpressing the 695 amine acid isoform of APP harboring two mutations (K670N, M671L) were soon generated. The mice develop age-dependent memory deficits and amyloid pathology, as well as elevated Aβ level [66]. Later a transgenic mouse using Thy-1 promoter to drive tau protein expression was produced which progressively develop many of the pathological hallmarks of AD including neurofibrillary tangles and abnormally hyperphosphorylated tau [67]. Apolipoprotein E 4 (ApoE4) polymorphism has been reported to be the major AD genetic risk factor [68], and ApoE4 transgenic mice were also established as AD model which display spatial learning and memory deficits [69]. Several APP/PS1 (with or without AD associated mutations) double transgenic mice were developed which displayed elevated Aβ generation, accelerated plaque development and memory deficits [70]. The APP/Tau double transgenic mice model was generated to study the interaction between Aβ and tau pathology in AD which develops both amyloid pathology and tau pathology [71]. A new transgenic mouse model combines APP, PS1, and tau mutations, was developed recently. The mice display more severe neuron loss and tau pathology including tau hyperphosphorylation, misfolding, and truncations [72].

Beyond the transgenic animal models, there are other widely used animal AD models, such as senescence-accelerated mice, toxin-induced lesion models, and neurotransmitter-based pharmacological models. Natural aging model and senescence-accelerated mice display some pathological phenomenon of AD [73, 74]. Direct intracerebral injection of Aβ causes accumulation of Aβ in brain and mediates oxidative stress, local cell loss, inflammation, and AD-like behavioral alterations [75]. Okadaic acid [76], ibotenic acid [77], colchicines [78], heavy metal [79], scopolamine [80], and NaN3 [81] were directly intracerebrally injected to induce AD-like neuronal lesion as well as learning and memory deficits. In addition to the animal model, many cell-based AD model were also established for mechanistic study and drug discovery. These models include Aβ incubation models, chemical-induced cell damage models, mutated APP transgenic cell models, and mutated tau transgenic cell models.

10.2.1.2 AD from View of Chinese Medicine

In CM theory, AD was covered in the disease of "Dementia" which was first used by a famous CM practitioner Zhang Jing-Yue in 1624. The definition of dementia is "a kind of mind disease which results from dysfunction of vital activities due to brain atrophy mainly manifested as dullness and stupidity" in CM theory. The key pathogenesis of dementia in CM is believed to include: (1) Deficiency of vital energy of the kidney, heart, and spleen; (2) Stagnation of blood and/or phlegm. Dementia could be classified into several subtypes based on their clinical patterns, such as *Gan-Shen Yin* Deficiency Syndrome, *Shen Essence* Deficiency Syndrome, *Qi* Stagnation and *Blood Stasis* Syndrome, *Pi-Shen Yang* Deficiency Syndrome, *Phelegm Turbid* Blocking *Orifice* Syndrome, and so on. Accordingly, CM formulas were prescribed aiming to improve *Shen-Qi* Deficiency, *Shen* Essence Deficiency, *Xin-Qi* Deficiency, Pi-Qi Deficiency, and Stagnation of *Blood* and *Phlegm*.

10.2.1.3 Neuroprotective Effect of CM-Derived Materials in the Experimental AD Models

CM-originated materials including formulas, single herb extracts, and single compounds have been widely tested on experimental AD models from cells to rodent. The main mechanisms of therapeutic actions involved in these CM for AD therapy are: (1) Anti-inflammatory; (2) Antioxidative stress; (3) Anti-apoptosis; (4) Induction of autophagy; (5) Regulating APP processing; (6) Inhibited Aβ accumulation; (7) Suppresses RAGE-dependent signaling, and so on.

Huperzine A is an alkaloid isolated from *Huperzia serrata* (Thunb) Trev, which is widely used in China to treat AD. Huperzine A significantly improved cognitive function in AD patients [82]. Timosaponin-B II is an extract from CM *Anemarrhena asphodeloides* Bunge, and has been administered as an antioxidant to alleviate AD pathology in a rodent AD model [83]. Indirubin is isolated from CM Indigo Naturalis and has been shown to inhibit two protein kinas involved in abnormal tau phosphorylation in AD [84]. It had been reported that EGb761 extracted from the leaf of *Ginkgo biloba* L can prevent and delay the progress of AD [85]. EGb761 is a mixture of terpenes, flavonoids, and organic acids, playing a substantial role in preventing apoptosis [86], oxidative stress [87], inflammation [88], and the Aβ fibril formation [89]. It has been reported that tenuifolin enhanced cholinergic neurotransmission, inhibited AchE activity, and decrease the secretion of Aβ [90]. Berberine is isolated from the CM herb *Coptis chinensis* Franch which can reduce Aβ secretion by altering APP processing in a way to shift from the amyloidogenic to nonamyloidogenic pathway [91]. Rhynchophylline extracted from *Uncaria hirsute* Havil could inhibit Aβ generation and prevention of Aβ fibril formation [92]. Timosaponin-B II could inhibit the BACE1 express and prevent Aβ accumulation. Notoginsenoside R1 can also inhibit Aβ accumulation [93]. For details of more CM-originated materials being tested in experimental AD models, please refer to Table 10.2.

10.2.2 Parkinson's Disease

PD is the second most common neurodegenerative disease characterized by progressive loss of dopaminergic neurons in the substantia nigra [94] and presence of intracytoplasmic inclusions called Lewy body in the cell body and neurites of affected neurons [95]. Genetic factors, oxidative stress, protein degradation deficits, mitochondria damages, metal toxicity, and environmental toxins are involved in the pathogenesis of PD. α-Synuclein (α-syn) is the primary component of Lewy bodies which is believed to be the critic event contributing to the development of PD. α-Syn induces oxidative stress [96], inflammatory [97] and affects autophagy pathway [98] in brain. The manifested broad spectrum of PD symptoms includes motor (resting tremor, bradykinesia, rigidity, and loss of postural reflexes) and nonmotor (sleep disturbances, constipation, anxiety, and depression) symptoms. Other clinical features include secondary motor symptoms, dysarthria, dysphagia, dystonia, freezing, festination, hypomimia, micrograohia, glabellar reflexes, sialorrhoea, shuffing gait. The current treatments for PD are mainly symptomatic to control the motor symptoms. Levodopa combined with carbidopa is the first-line drug for PD which can help to control the symptoms effectively; however, levodopa cannot slow down the neurodegeneration process and long-term effects of levodopa are disappointing. There is a need to identify new therapeutic intervention to prevent the dopaminergic neuron degeneration.

10.2.2.1 Experiment PD Models

Many experimental models have been developed to study the disease mechanism and test therapeutic interventions. These models can be divided into two types:

Table 10.2 Pharmacological effects of CM on AD and PD

Pharmacological effects of CM on AD models						
Formula/extract/compounds	CM herbs	Model	Drug administration protocol	Pharmacological activity	Mechanism of action	Ref.
70 % ethanol extract of Huanglian jiedu Decoction (黃連解毒湯)	*Coptischinensis* Franch (黃連), *Scutellaria baicalensis* Georgi (黃芩), *Phellodendron chinense* C.K. Schneid (黃柏) and *Gardenia jasminoides* J. Ellis (梔子)	Senescence-accelerated mouse (SAMP8); N2a-SwedAPP cells	p.o. at 5 g/kg/day for 30 days; N2a-SwedAPP cells treated with 0.3–50 μg/ml extract for 48 h	Downregulated caMKII α and upregulated AMF and AMFR in the hippocampus; reduce Aβ production in N2a-SwedAPP cells	Affect caMKIIα and AMFR expression; affect APP procession	[120–122]
80 % ethanol extract of Qingxue-dan (清血丹)	*Scutellaria baicalensis* Georgi (黃芩), *Coptis chinensis* Franch (黃連), *Phellodendron chinense* C.K. Schneid (黃柏), *Gardenia jasminoides* J. Ellis (梔子) and *Rheum officinale* Baill (大黃)	PC12 and BV-2 cell treat with Aβ oligomer	Cells treated with 0.1–100 μg/ml extract for 24 h in the presence of 1 μM Aβ oligomer	Increase in cell viability Reducing nitric oxide (NO), tumor necrosis factor-α(TNF-α), interleukin-1β(IL-β) and IL-6 production	Anti-inflammatory	[123]
Distilled water extract of Shenmai san (生脈散)	*Panax ginseng* C.A. Mey (人蔘), *Ophiopogon japonicus* (Thunb.) Ker Gawl (麥冬), *Schisandra chinensis* (Turcz.) Baill (五味子)	PC12 cells treated with H_2O_2 for 30 min	Cells treated with 0.16–0.66 μg/ml extract for 24 h in the presence of H_2O_2	Increase in cell viability Decrease in ROS level	Antioxidative stress	[124]
Distilled water extract of Buyang Huanwu Decoction (補陽還五湯)	*Angelica dahurica* (Hoffm.) Benth (白芷), *Paeonia anomala* L. (赤芍), *Ligusticum sinense cv. chuanxiong* (川芎), *Prunus persica* (L.) Batsch (桃仁), *Carthamus tinctorius* L. (紅花) and *Amynthas aspergillus* (地龍)	Scopolamine injected Mice model (4 mg/kg, i.p.)	p.o. at 6.65 g/kg twice a day for 7 days before ischemia	Reduced injury in hippocampal CA1 region; Decreased TUNEL-positive neurons number	Anti-apoptosis	[117]

(continued)

Table 10.2 (continued)

Pharmacological effects of CM on AD models						
Formula/extract/compounds	CM herbs	Model	Drug administration protocol	Pharmacological activity	Mechanism of action	Ref.
The supercritical CO_2 and water extracts of FuLing-BaiZhu-DangGui (FBD) (茯苓白朮當歸)	*Wolfiporia extensa* (Peck) Ginns (茯苓), *Atractylodes japonica* Koidz (蒼朮), *Angelica sinensis* (Oliv.) Diels (當歸)	Scopolamine injected ICR mice model (4 mg/kg, i.p.)	p.o. 200 and 600 mg/kg daily for 6 days	Improve scopolamine induced memory deficit	Brain acetylcholinesterase (AChE) and circulating butyrylcholinesterase inhibition	[125]
A standard extract of ginkgo (EGb761)	*Ginkgo biloba* L. (銀杏葉)	TgCRND8 Tg mice	p.o. 69 mg/kg per daily for 5 months	Improved the cognitive function, attenuated the synaptic degeneration, inhibited microglial inflammatory activation	Anti-inflammatory, induction of autophagy, anti-amyloidgenic	[126]
Water extract of green tea	*Camellia sinensis* (L.) Kuntze (綠茶)	Primary mouse hippocampal neuron culture treated with Aβ	Cells treated with 10 μg/ml extract for 24 h	Reduced neuronal apoptosis	ROS scavenging	[127]
Compound K	*Panax ginseng* C.A. Mey (人蔘)	Primary culture of mouse astrocytes	Cells treated with 1–50 μM compound K for 18 h	Promotes Aβ clearance	Activates autophagy by inhibiting phosphorylation of mTOR	[128]
Huperzine	*Huperzia serrata* (Thunb) Trev (蛇足石杉)	PC12 cells treat with Aβ; Permanent ligation of the common carotid arteries	Cell preincubated with Huperzine for 2 h before adding Aβ25–35; p.o. at 0.1 mg/kg, twice per day for 18 days	Promotes cell survival; restored the decrease in acetylcholinesterase activity, improved cognitive function	Antioxidative stress, Anti- apoptosis, AChE inhibition, mitochondrial protection	[129–133]

(continued)

Table 10.2 (continued)

Pharmacological effects of CM on AD models						
Formula/extract/compounds	CM herbs	Model	Drug administration protocol	Pharmacological activity	Mechanism of action	Ref.
Evodiamine	*Tetradium ruticarpum* (A. Juss.) T.G. Hartley (吳茱萸)	SAMF8, APPswe/PS1ΔE9 transgenic mouse models	p.o. at 50 and 100 mg/kg daily for 4 weeks	Reversed the inhibition of glucose uptake; decreased the expression of IL-1β, IL-6, TNF-α, and COX-2	Anti-inflammatory, restore glucose uptake	[134]
Tetramethylpyrazine	*Ligusticum sinense cv. chuanxiong* (川芎)	H_2O_2-induced apoptosis in PC12 cells	Cells were preincubated with TMP for 4 h and H_2O_2 was added to the medium for an additional 12 h	Prevents H_2O_2-induced cell death	Anti-apoptosis	[135, 136]
Berberine	*Coptis chinensis* Franch (黃連)	TgCRND8 mice	i.g. 25–100 mg/kg per day for 4 months	Attenuate Aβ deposits, tau hyperphosphorylation and gliosis	Regulating APP processing	[137]
Uncariarhynchophylla	*Uncaria hirsute* Havil (鈎藤)	Aβ induced neurotoxicity in PC12 cells model	Cells preincubated with Uncaria rhynchophylla for 2 h and Aβ added to the medium for an additional 24 h	Decreased Aβ-induced cell death, intracellular calcium overloading, and tau hyperphosphorylation in PC12 cells	Anti-apoptosis, inhibitory and destabilizing effects on Aβ fibrils	[138, 139]
Liquiritin	*Glycyrrhiza uralensis* Fisch (乾草)	PC12 cells grown in serum starvation DMEM for 12 h	Dissolved in DMSO and diluted in DMEM 5–100 μM treatment for 24 h	Promotes neurite outgrowth	Overexpression of neural related genes	[140]

(continued)

Table 10.2 (continued)

Pharmacological effects of CM on AD models						
Formula/extract/compounds	CM herbs	Model	Drug administration protocol	Pharmacological activity	Mechanism of action	Ref.
Baicalin	*Scutellaria baicalensis* Georgi (黃芩)	Aβ injected rats model; Aβ induced neurotoxicity in SH-SY5Y and BV-2 cells	i.p. 50–200 mg/kg baicalin; Cells incubated with baicalin at 0.1–10 μM for 2 h before Aβ treatment	Prevented Aβ-induced learning and memory deficit; reduced neuron toxicity; attenuated the inflammation	Anti-apoptosis, antioxidative stress, Anti-inflammatory	[141–143]
Icariin	*Epimedium brevicornu* Maxim (淫羊藿)	Aβ induced neurotoxicity in PC12 cells; CORT caused apoptosis in primary hypothalamic neurons	Cells were pretreated with 2.5, 5, 10, 10 μM concentrations of icariin for 30 min, followed by exposure to Aβ	Deceased Aβ induced cytotoxicity, inhibited tau hyperphosphorylation; Decreased CORT-induced cell death	Inhibits GSK-3β; Activates the PI3-K/Akt pathway	[144, 145]
Puerarin	*Pueraria montana* var. *Lobata* (Willd.) (葛根)	Aβ induced neurotoxicity in PC12 cells model	Dissolved in DMEM 24 h treatment 0.1–1000 μM	Prevent Aβ induced cell death	Activates PI3K/Akt signaling pathway	[146]
Forsythiaside	*Forsythia suspense* (Thunb.) Vahl (連翹)	SAMP8 mice	p.o. at 60, 120, 240 mg/kg daily for 6 days	Attenuates cognitive impairment	Antioxidative stress, anti-apoptosis, and anti-inflammation	[147]
Osthole	*Cnidium monnieri* (L.) Cusson (蛇床子)	Aβ injected rats model; Aβ induced neurotoxicity in SH-SY5Y cells	i.p. with osthole (12.5 mg/kg or 25.0 mg/kg) once a day for 14 days	Improved learning and memory impairment and increased synaptic plasticity	Enhances CREB Phosphorylation and decreases BACE1 level	[148, 149]
Ferulic acid	*Ferula asafoetida* L. (阿魏)	Aβ injection induced cognitive deficits in rats	p.o. 50, 100 mg/kg for 2 months	Attenuates cognitive impairment	Antioxidative stress, AChE inhibition	[150]
Schisandrone	*Schisandra chinensis* (Turcz.) Baill (五味子)	Aβ injection injected mice model	p.o.15, 150 ug/kg for 5 days	Ameliorates learning and memory deficits	Antioxidative stress, ChE inhibition	[151]

(continued)

Table 10.2 (continued)

Pharmacological effects of CM on AD models						
Formula/extract/compounds	CM herbs	Model	Drug administration protocol	Pharmacological activity	Mechanism of action	Ref.
Notoginsenoside	*Panax notoginseng* (Burkill) F.H. Chen ex C.H. Chow (三七)	APP/PS1 double transgenic mouse model	p.o. 5 mg/(kg d), 25 mg/(kg d) for 3 months	Ameliorated the cognitive impairment and increased AChE expression	Increased insulin degrading enzyme expression and inhibited Aβ accumulation	[93]
Timosaponin	*Anemarrhena asphodeloides* Bunge (知母)	Rat retina pretreated with the FeCl3	i.v. 6 mg/kg for 14 days	Inhibited the upregulation of BACE1 and reduced the overproduction of β-CTF and Aβ in rat retina induced by FeCl3	Antioxidative stress	[152]
Tenuigenin	*Polygala tenuifolia* Willd (遠志)	COS-7 cells transfected with APP695 cDNA	Cells treated with 0.5–2 μM Tenuigenin	Inhibited Aβ secretion	Inhibition of the beta-site APP cleaving enzyme	[153]
Gastrodin	*Gastrodia elata* Blume (天麻)	Tg2576 transgenic	p.o. 60 mg/kg for 15 days	Alleviates memory deficits and reduces neuropathology	Anti-inflammatory, reduced iNOS, COX-2, TNF-α, and IL-1β level	[154]
Geniposide	*jasminoides* J. Ellis (梔子)	mPrP-APPswe/PS1dE9 AD transgenic mice	p.o. 25 mg/kg/day for 3 months	Attenuated impaired synaptic plasticity as well as learning and memory defects, reduced cerebral Aβ accumulation	suppresses RAGE-dependent signaling and inflammation	[155]

(continued)

Table 10.2 (continued)

Pharmacological effects of CM on AD models						
Formula/extract/compounds	CM herbs	Model	Drug administration protocol	Pharmacological activity	Mechanism of action	Ref.
Triptolide	*Tripterygium wilfordii* Hook (雷公藤)	5XFAD mice	i.p. 20 μg/kg for 8 weeks	Enhanced spatial learning performances, and attenuated Aβ pathology in the brain	Antioxidative stress Anti-inflammatory	[156]
Curcumin	*Curcuma longa* L. (薑黃)	APP/PS1 double transgenic mice	p.o. 160 ppm and 1000 ppm for 6 months	Attenuated cognitive impairment and inhibited the generation of Aβ	Inhibits PI3K/Akt/mTOR signaling pathway	[157]
Pharmacological effects of CM on PD models						
80 % ethanol extract of Qingxue-dan (清血丹)	*Scutellaria baicalensis* Georgi (黃芩), *Coptis chinensis* Franch (黃連), *Phellodendron chinense* C.K. Schneid (黃柏), *Gardenia jasminoides* J. Ellis (梔子) and *Rheum officinale* Baill (大黃)	PC12 cell treat with 100 μM 6–OHDA	Cells pretreated with 0.1–100 μg/ml of CHD for 3 h before 100 μM 6-OHDA treatment for 6 h	Prevented ROS-mediated neuronal cell death	Antioxidative stress Anti-apoptosis	[113]
Distilled water extract of Shenmai san (生脈散)	*Panax ginseng* C.A. Mey (人蔘), *Ophiopogon japonicus* (Thunb.) Ker Gawl (麥冬), *Schisandra chinensis* (Turcz.) Baill (五味子)	PC12 cells treated with H_2O_2 in serum-free DMEM for 30 min	Cells treated with 0.16–0.66 μg/ml extract for 2 h and incubated with H_2O_2 for 24 h	Prevented ROS-mediated neuronal cell death	Antioxidative stress	[124]
Extract of Cassiae semen (COE)	*Senna tora* (L.) Roxb (覺明子)	PC12 cells treat 100 μM 6-OHDA	Cells pretreated with 0.1–50 μg/ml of COE before 6-OHDA treatment	Prevented ROS-mediated neuronal cell death	Antioxidative stress	[158]

(continued)

Table 10.2 (continued)

Pharmacological effects of CM on AD models						
Formula/extract/compounds	CM herbs	Model	Drug administration protocol	Pharmacological activity	Mechanism of action	Ref.
A standard extract of ginkgo (EGb761)	*Ginkgo biloba* L. (銀杏葉)	MPTP-injected mice model	p.o. 40 and 80 mg/kg for 7 days after the last MPTP injection	Attenuated loss of striatal dopamine levels and tyrosine hydroxylase immunostaining, improved impairment of locomotion	Antioxidative stress	[159]
Gingseng total saponins	*Panax ginseng* C.A. Mey (人蔘)	MPTP treated PC12 cells	Cells pretreated with 0.1–1.5 mg/ml saponins for 1 h before MPTP treatment for 12 h	Prevented ROS-mediated neuronal cell death	Anti-apoptosis	[160]
Corynoxine and Corynoxine B	Ramulus *Uncaria rhynchophylla* (鉤藤)	α-syn over expression in N2a cells	Cells treated with 5–25 μM compounds for 24 h	Induces autophagy	mTOR-dependent and mTOR-independent	[161, 162]
Puerarin	*Pueraria montana* var. *Lobata* (Willd.) (葛根)	Rotenone treated rat and SH-SY5Y cell model	p.o. 50 mg/Kg, 100 mg/Kg for 7 days; Cells treated with 50–150 μM puerarin	Increased cell viability, decreased ROS level Enhanced degradation of aggregated protein	Antioxidative stress, anti-apoptosis	[163]
Tubuloside B	*Cistanche deserticola* Y.C. Ma (肉蓯蓉)	MPP+ treat PC12 cells,	Cells treated with 10–100 μM tubuloside for 48–72 with MPP+	Prevented ROS-mediated neuronal cell death	Antioxidative stress	[164]

(continued)

Table 10.2 (continued)

Pharmacological effects of CM on AD models						
Formula/extract/compounds	CM herbs	Model	Drug administration protocol	Pharmacological activity	Mechanism of action	Ref.
Phenylethanoid glycosides (PhGs)	*Cistanche deserticola* Y.C. Ma (肉苁蓉)	MPTP-lesioned C57mice	p.o, PhGs 10, 50 mg/kg for 2 weeks	Improved impaired motor function, rescued decreased striatal Dopamine levels	Facilitates striatal DA release	[165]
Ginsenoside Rb1	*Panax ginseng* C.A. Mey (人蔘)	6-OHDA-based SH-SY5Y cells	Cells treated with 10, 30, 100 μM Rb1 for 24 h	Prevented ROS-mediated neuronal cell death, Restored mitochondrial membrane potential, increased energy production	Antioxidative stress mitochondrial protection	[166, 167]
Ginsenoside Re	*Panax ginseng* C.A. Mey (人蔘)	MPTP-lesioned C57mice	i.g. 6.5, 13, 26 mg/kg/day for 13 days	Increase TH-positive neurons, inhibiting the activation of caspase3	Anti-apoptosis	[168]
Salvianolic acid B	*Salvia miltiorrhiza* Bunge (丹参)	6-OHDA-based SH-SY5Y cells	Cells pretreated with 2–10 μM Sal B 1 h before 100 μM 6-OHDA treatment for 24 h	Prevented ROS-mediated neuronal cell death	Antioxidative stress, anti-apoptosis	[169]
Tanshinone I	*Salvia miltiorrhiza* Bunge (丹参)	LPS-induced BV-2 microglia cell model, MPTP-lesioned C57 mice	Cell pretreated with 1–20 μM Tanshinone I before LPS treatment; p.o. 5–10 mg/kg for 7 days	Suppressed microglia activation and prevented nigrostriatal dopaminergic neurodegeneration	Anti-inflammation	[170]

(continued)

Table 10.2 (continued)

Pharmacological effects of CM on AD models						
Formula/extract/compounds	CM herbs	Model	Drug administration protocol	Pharmacological activity	Mechanism of action	Ref.
Baicalein	*Scutellaria baicalensis* Georgi (黃芩)	MPTP-lesioned C57 mice, α-syn aggregation	p.o. Baicalein (5, 10 mg/kg per day) for 14 days, 1–100 μM incubation	Inhibited the activation of microglia and astrocytes in substantia nigra	Anti-inflammation	[171–173]
Baicalin	*Scutellaria baicalensis* Georgi (黃芩)	Rotenone-induced Wistar rats model	i.g. 78 mg/kg per day for 8 weeks	Inhibited iron accumulation in different brain regions	Reduce the toxicity of metals	[174, 175]
Bilobalide	*Ginkgo biloba* L. (銀杏葉)	6-OHDA-based rat models	i.p. 5, 10, 20 mg/kg once a day for 7 days	Inhibited loss of TH-positive neurons, decreased the activation of NF-κB	Anti-apoptosis, anti-inflammation	[176]
Lyceum barbarum polysaccharides	*Lycium barbarum* L. (枸杞子)	PC12 cells incubated with 75 μM 6-OHDA for 24 h	Cells were treated with 100–600 μM LBP for 24 h	Prevented ROS-mediated neuronal cell death	Antioxidative stress, anti-inflammation	[114]
Berberine	*Coptis chinensis* Franch (黃連)	MPTP i.p. induced C57 mice model	p.o. 20 mg/Kg and 50 mg/Kg for 5 weeks	Prevented nigrostriatal dopaminergic neuronal loss, suppressed hippocampal apoptosis, and improved short-time memory	Anti-apoptosis, anti-inflammation	[177]
Tetramethylpyrazine (TMP)	*Ligusticum sinense cv. chuanxiong* (川芎)	MPTP i.p. induced mice model	i.p. 3–30 mg/Kg for 2 weeks	Inhibited the synthesis of cytokines, recovered the dopamine deficits and improved the behavioral performance	Antioxidative stress Anti-inflammation	[178]

(continued)

Table 10.2 (continued)

Pharmacological effects of CM on AD models						
Formula/extract/compounds	CM herbs	Model	Drug administration protocol	Pharmacological activity	Mechanism of action	Ref.
Quercetin	*Quercus dentata* Thunb (槲皮)	PC12 cells treated with 100 μM of 6-OHDA for 24 h	Pretreated for 8 h with 10 μM quercetin before 6-OHDA treatment	Prevented ROS-mediated neuronal cell death Upregulated the TH, ion transport and anti-apoptotic genes	Anti-apoptosis, regulates gene expression	[179]
Curcumin	*Curcuma longa* L. (薑黃)	SH-SY5Ycells treated with 25 μM of 6-OHDA for 24 h	Cells treated with 5–20μM Curcumin 30 min before 6-OHDA 6-OHDA treatment	Prevented 6-OHDA-mediated cell death, Reduced ROS, inhibited α-syn aggregation	Anti-inflammation Antioxidative stress Inhibit fibrillation	[180, 181]
Notoginsenoside-Rg1	*Panax notoginseng* (Burkill) F.H. Chen ex C.H. Chow (三七)	SH-SY5Ycells treated with 50 μM of 6-OHDA for 24 h	Cells pretreated with 20 μM notoginsenoside R2 for 24h	Prevented 6-OHDA-mediated cell death, Reduced ROS	Anti-inflammatory Anti-apoptosis	[182]
Resveratrol	*Fallopia japonica* (Houtt.) Ronse Decr (虎杖)	MPTP i.p. induced mice model; primary fibroblast cultures from patients	p.o. 10–100 mg/kg for 21 days; Cells pretreated with 25 μM resveratrol for 24 h	Reduced glial activation, decreased IL-6 and TNF-α levels; Improved mitochondrial activity and energy homeostasis	Anti-inflammation, activation of AMPK, SIRT1, and PGC-1α	[183, 184]

toxin-induced models and genetic models. The toxin-induced models aim to reproduce the behavioral abnormality and neurodegeneration features of PD. 6-Hydroxydopamine (6-OHDA) is the first identified and still widely used classic PD toxin [99]. 6-OHDA does not cross the blood–brain barrier, and has to be directly injected into the substantianigra pars (SNpc) compacta, striatum, or the medial forebrain bundle (MFB) parts to induce oxidative stress, inflammation, and destroy catecholaminergic neurons [100]. After getting into the cells via dopamine transporter, 6-OHDA accumulates in the mitochondria where it inhibits complex I activity and leads to oxidative stress. By killing TH-positive neuron, 6-OHDA causes striatum-nigra system dysfunction and behavioral abnormalities. Other neurotoxins such as 1-methyl-1,2,3,6-tetrahydropiridine (MPTP) [101], rotenone [102], and paraqua [103] are also developed to induce PD lesion in animals via similar toxic mechanism.

The discovery of PD-associated genes is particularly exciting because these discoveries have prompted our understanding toward the pathogenesis of PD and the development of new models of PD. α-Synuclein coding gene *SNCA* was the first gene to be linked to familiar form of PD and three point mutations (A30P, A53T, E46 K) are regarded as causative to PD. A number of *SNCA* transgenic mice have been established using a variety of promoters, such as TH promoter [104], PDGFβ promoter [105], Thy1 promoter [106], and mPrP promoter [107]. These *SNCA* transgenic mice developed PD-related pathological features including intraneuronal inclusions, dopamine reduction, TH-positive neuron loss, and motor function impairments. Recently some scientists inject *SNCA* AAV virus or α-synuclein fibrils into striatum or substantial nigra region to establish PD models which display typical PD-associated phenotypes including intraneuronal inclusion, TH neuron degeneration, and impaired motor function. *Leucine rich repeat kinase 2* (*LRRK2*) gene mutations have been associated with both inherited form and sporadic form of PD thus triggers wide attention [108]. BAC transgenic mice overexpressing G2019S and R1441G mutant LRRK2 protein have been widely used as PD animal model. However, despite reduced dopamine level and impaired neuritis growth were reported in these mice, no obvious signs of neurodegeneration, intraneuronal inclusion formation, and motor function impairment were observed [109, 110]. Mutations in *Parkin*, *DJ1*, and *PINK1* genes have been linked to familiar recessive forms of PD. KO of these genes recapitulated specific aspects of PD pathology such as mitochondria dysfunction, however none of the models generate the neuronal degeneration phenotype [111].

10.2.2.2 PD from View of Chinese Medicine

The earliest description of PD symptoms can be found in the classic traditional Chinese Medicine book, "Yellow Emperor Canon of Inner Medicine". In the book, the PD-likely symptom is described as "*wind* refers to the symptoms of shaking and dizziness, resulting from the dysfunction of *Gan* and the symptoms of stiffness and spasm result from *wind* or *Dampness*". According to CM theory, PD can be classified into several subtypes based on the clinical patterns: *Qi stagnation* and *Blood Stasis Syndrome*, *Qi-blood Deficiency Syndrome*, *Gan-Shen Yin Deficiency Syndrome, Phlegm Stagnation Syndrome*, and *Shen-Yang Deficiency Syndrome.* Accordingly, treatment strategies are to "calm the *gan-wind*", "dissipating *phlegm* for resuscitation", and "nourish the *Gan-Shen Yin deficiency*". "Tianma gouteng decoction" is a widely used CM formula to calm the *gan-wind* for PD treatment. "*Jia Wei Liu Jun Zi Tang* [*JWLJZT*]" is an ancient formula to tonify the *Spleen-stomach Qi* and has been shown to improve the nonmotor function of PD patients [112].

10.2.2.3 Neuroprotective Effect of CM-Derived Materials in the Experimental PD Models

There are many reports showing that CM can relieve the clinical symptoms of PD, implying that CM may improve the motor function of the patients and slow down the DA neuron degeneration. The neuroprotective effects of CM-originated materials have been tested on the PD models. The mechanisms of therapeutic actions involved in these CM-originated materials for PD therapy include inhibition of apoptosis, inhibition of oxidative stress, inhibition of neural immune and inflammatory responses, improving mitochondrial energy metabolism, inhibition of abnormal protein aggregation, and induction of autophagy. For example, Extract from Qingxue-dan has been shown to exert neuroprotective effects by inhibiting the release of proinflammatory molecules, ROS, and regulation of Bcl-2 family proteins [113]. *Lycium barbarum* polysaccharides (LBP), extracted from the fruits of *Lycium barbarum* L, have been shown to prevent 6-OHDA-induced apoptosis in PC12 cells through inhibited the ROS-NO pathway [114]. Baicalein is a flavonoid isolated from the *Scutellaria baicalensis* Georgi which has been reported to mitigate the behavioral abnormality in the animal model of PD through inhibiting the activation of astrocytes and microglia in substantia nigra. For details of more CM-originated materials being tested in experimental PD models, please refer to Table 10.2.

10.3 Conclusion

CM has been widely used for treating stroke, AD, and PD in Asia from ancient to today. Though accumulating evidence suggests its efficacy in clinic practice, several concerns impair the enthusiasm toward more wide use of CM: the standardization of clinical trials, the quality control of CM and the molecular mechanism of pharmacological action. In this chapter, the experimental data showing the efficacy of CM in the neurological diseases models and the possible molecular mechanism are summarized and discussed. By providing experimental data and uncovering underlying mechanism, the mystery of CM will be better understood.

Numerous studies reported the protective effect of CM-originated materials on the stroke, AD, and PD models. Among the mechanisms being revealed, antioxidative stress and anti-inflammation are the most common mechanism underlying the neuroprotectivity. Oxidative stress and inflammation are critic events during these diseases course. The CM-originated materials either serve as ROS scavengers, or regulate cellular antioxidant system to prevent the oxidative stress, and regulate the secretion of proinflammation cytokine release to inhibit inflammation. Other mechanisms including neurotropic effect, mitochondria biogenesis, autophagy induction, anti-iron toxicity, restoring ion homeostasis are also reported to be involved in the neuroprotection. However, it has to be admitted that the mechanisms underlying the neuroprotectivity of CM-originated materials are still not fully understood.

The extracts from formulas and single herbs, as well as single compounds from CM are extensively tested in these neurological diseases models. It is always easier to investigate the molecular mechanism of single compounds compared with extract that may contain thousands of compounds. However, the CM is administrated to patients as extract not single compounds. The pharmacological activity of extract may lose once the mixture was separated into single compounds and this happens very often. It is therefore better to test pharmacological effects of both extracts and representative compounds, especially on animal diseases models. Considering that multiple factors and pathways are involved in the complex disease course, mixture of compounds that target at different pathways may lead to a better protection compared with single compounds. Based on the accumulating evidence revealing neuroprotective effect of CM-originated materials, we are optimistic that CM can be a potential source for drug discovery against neurological diseases including stroke, AD, and PD.

Acknowledgments This work was supported by grants from Macao Science and Technology Development Fund (FDCT_No.022/2015/A1) and China National Science Foundation (NSFC_No.31500831) awarded to Jia-hong Lu.

References

1. Liu T, Li X, Zou ZY, Li C. The prevalence and determinants of using traditional chinese medicine among middle-aged and older chinese adults: results from the china health and retirement longitudinal study. J Am Med Dir Assoc. 2015.
2. Rajendran PR, Thompson RE, Reich SG. The use of alternative therapies by patients with Parkinson's disease. Neurology. 2001;57(5):790–4.
3. Mozaffarian D, Benjamin EJ, Go AS, Arnett DK, Blaha MJ, Cushman M, et al. Heart disease and stroke statistics-2015 update: a report from the american heart association. Circulation. 2015;131(4):e29.
4. Junhua Z, Menniti-Ippolito F, Xiumei G, Firenzuoli F, Boli Z, Massari M, et al. Complex traditional chinese medicine for poststroke motor dysfunction a systematic review. Stroke. 2009;40(8):2797–804.

5. Traystman RJ. Animal models of focal and global cerebral ischemia. ILAR J. 2003;44(2):85–95.
6. Endres M DU. Neuroprotective strategies in animal and in vitro-models of neuronal damage: ischemiia and stroke. In: Alzheimer C, editor. Molecular and cellular biology of neuroprotection in CNS. New York: Kluwer Academic and Landes Bioscience; 2003. 513:455–7.
7. Myers RE, Yamaguchi SI. Nervous system effects of cardiac arrest in monkeys: preservation of vision. Arch Neurol. 1977;34(2):65–74.
8. Nemoto EM, Bleyaert AL, Stezoski S, Moossy J, Rao GR, Safar P. Global brain ischemia: a reproducible monkey model. Stroke. 1977;8(5):558–64.
9. Brint S, Jacewicz M, Kiessling M, Tanabe J, Pulsinelli W. Focal brain ischemia in the rat: methods for reproducible neocortical infarction using tandem occlusion of the distal middle cerebral and ipsilateral commoncarotid arteries. J Cereb Blood Flow Metab. 1988;8(4):474–85.
10. De Ley G, Weyne J, Demeester G, Stryckmans K, Goethals P, Leusen I. Streptokinase treatment versus calcium overload blockade in experimental thromboembolic stroke. Stroke. 1989;20(3):357–61.
11. Clark WM, Madden KP, Rothlein R, Zivin JA. Reduction of central nervous system ischemic injury in rabbits using leukocyte adhesion antibody treatment. Stroke. 1991;22(7):877–83.
12. Ames A 3rd, Wright RL, Kowada M, Thurston JM, Majno G. Cerebral ischemia. II. The no-reflow phenomenon. Am J Pathol. 1968;52(2):437–53.
13. Endres M, Namura S, Shimizu-Sasamata M, Waeber C, Zhang L, Gomez-Isla T, et al. Attenuation of delayed neuronal death after mild focal ischemia in mice by inhibition of the caspase family. J Cereb Blood Flow Metab. 1998;18(3):238–47.
14. MacLellan CL, Silasi G, Auriat AM, Colbourne F. Rodent models of intracerebral hemorrhage. Stroke. 2010;41(10 suppl 1):S95–8.
15. Belayev L. Blood injection intracerebral hemorrhage mouse model. In: Chen J, Xu Z, Xu X-M, Zhang J, editors. Animal models of acute neurological injuries. Humana Press; 2009. p. 349–57.
16. Tasca CI, Dal-Cim T, Cimarosti H. In vitro oxygen–glucose deprivation to study ischemic cell death. Neuronal cell death. Springer; 2015. p. 197–210.
17. Newcomb-Fernandez JK, Zhao X, Pike BR, Wang KK, Kampfl A, Beer R, et al. Concurrent assessment of calpain and caspase-3 activation after oxygen–glucose deprivation in primary septo-hippocampal cultures. J Cereb Blood Flow Metab. 2001;21(11):1281–94.
18. Fernandez-Lopez D, Martinez-Orgado J, Casanova I, Bonet B, Leza JC, Lorenzo P, et al. Immature rat brain slices exposed to oxygen–glucose deprivation as an in vitro model of neonatal hypoxic-ischemic encephalopathy. J Neurosci Methods. 2005;145(1–2):205–12.
19. Gong X, Sucher NJ. Stroke therapy in traditional Chinese medicine (TCM): prospects for drug discovery and development. Trends Pharmacol Sci. 1999;20(5):191–6.
20. Adams JD, Lien EJ. Traditional Chinese medicine: scientific basis for its use. Royal Society of Chemistry; 2013.
21. Wang P-R, Wang J-S, Yang M-H, Kong L-Y. Neuroprotective effects of Huang-Lian-Jie-Du-Decoction on ischemic stroke rats revealed by 1H NMR metabolomics approach. J Pharm Biomed Anal. 2014;88:106–16.
22. Yun SP, Jung WS, Park SU, Moon SK, Ko CN, Cho KH, et al. Anti-hypertensive effect of chunghyul-dan (qingxue-dan) on stroke patients with essential hypertension. Am J Chin Med. 2005;33(03):357–64.
23. Xuejiang W, Magara T, Konishi T. Prevention and repair of cerebral ischemia-reperfusion injury by Chinese herbal medicine, shengmai san, in rats. Free Radical Res. 1999;31(5):449–55.
24. Guo Q, Zhong M, Xu H, Mao X, Zhang Y, Lin N. A systems biology perspective on the molecular mechanisms underlying the therapeutic effects of Buyang Huanwu Decoction on ischemic stroke. Rejuvenation Res. 2015.

25. Kim H. Neuroprotective herbs for stroke therapy in traditional eastern medicine. Neurol Res. 2005;27(3):287–301.
26. Sucher NJ. Insights from molecular investigations of traditional Chinese herbal stroke medicines: implications for neuroprotective epilepsy therapy. Epilepsy Behav. 2006;8 (2):350–62.
27. Gaire BP, Kim YO, Jin ZH, Park J, Choi H, Bu Y, et al. Neuroprotective effect of Scutellaria baicalensis flavones against global ischemic model in rats. J Nepal Pharm Assoc. 2015;27 (1):1–8.
28. Zhang Y, Wang X, Wang X, Xu Z, Liu Z, Ni Q, et al. Protective effect of flavonoids from Scutellaria baicalensis Georgi on cerebral ischemia injury. J Ethnopharmacol. 2006;108 (3):355–60.
29. Chen Y, Tsai Y-H, Tseng S-H. The potential of tetrandrine as a protective agent for ischemic stroke. Molecules. 2011;16(9):8020–32.
30. Sun X, Chan LN, Gong X, Sucher NJ. N-methyl-D-aspartate receptor antagonist activity in traditional Chinese stroke medicines. Neurosignals. 2003;12(1):31–8.
31. Lao CJ, Lin JG, Kuo JS, Chiang SY, Chen SC, Liao ET, et al. Effect of Salvia Miltiorrhiza Bunge on cerebral infarct in ischemia-reperfusion injured rats. Am J Chin Med. 2003;31 (2):191–200.
32. Suk K, Kim SY, Leem K, Kim YO, Park SY, Hur J, et al. Neuroprotection by methanol extract of Uncaria rhynchophylla against global cerebral ischemia in rats. Life Sci. 2002;70 (21):2467–80.
33. G-q Zheng, Cheng W, Wang Y, X-m Wang, S-z Zhao, Zhou Y, et al. Ginseng total saponins enhance neurogenesis after focal cerebral ischemia. J Ethnopharmacol. 2011;133(2):724–8.
34. Cheon SY, Cho KJ, Lee JE, Kim HW, Lee SK, Kim HJ, et al. Cerebroprotective effects of red ginseng extract pretreatment against ischemia-induced oxidative stress and apoptosis. Int J Neurosci. 2013;123(4):269–77.
35. Zhang Z, Peng D, Zhu H, Wang X. Experimental evidence of Ginkgo biloba extract EGB as a neuroprotective agent in ischemia stroke rats. Brain Res Bull. 2012;87(2):193–8.
36. Xie Y, Zhang B, Zhang Y. Protective effects of Acanthopanax polysaccharides on cerebral ischemia–reperfusion injury and its mechanisms. Int J Biol Macromol. 2015;72:946–50.
37. Wu K-J, Hsieh M-T, Wu C-R, Wood WG, Chen Y-F. Green tea extract ameliorates learning and memory deficits in ischemic rats via its active component polyphenol epigallocatechin-3-gallate by modulation of oxidative stress and neuroinflammation. Evid Based Complement Altern Med. 2012;2012.
38. Tao Y-w, Wang Y, Lai B-l, Tian G-y, Feng J-p, Su J-x. Protective effect of polysaccharide from the root of Rhizoma Corydalis on focal ischemic cerebral infarct induced by middle cerebral artery occlusion in rats. J Med Plants Res. 2013;7(4):140–7.
39. Choi YB, Kim YI, Lee KS, Kim BS. Protective effect of epigallocatechin gallate on brain damage after transient middle cerebral artery occlusion in rats. Brain Res. 2004;1019(1):47–54.
40. Yoshikawa T, Akiyoshi Y, Susumu T, Tokado H, Fukuzaki K, Nagata R, et al. Ginsenoside Rb1 reduces neurodegeneration in the peri-infarct area of a thromboembolic stroke model in non-human primates. J Pharmacol Sci. 2008;107(1):32–40.
41. Zhu J, Jiang Y, Wu L, Lu T, Xu G, Liu X. Suppression of local inflammation contributes to the neuroprotective effect of ginsenoside Rb1 in rats with cerebral ischemia. Neuroscience. 2012;202:342–51.
42. X-k Tu, W-z Yang, S-s Shi, C-h Wang, C-m Chen. Neuroprotective effect of baicalin in a rat model of permanent focal cerebral ischemia. Neurochem Res. 2009;34(9):1626–34.
43. Gao L, Ji X, Song J, Liu P, Yan F, Gong W, et al. Puerarin protects against ischemic brain injury in a rat model of transient focal ischemia. Neurol Res. 2009;31(4):402–6.
44. Lee W-T, Lin M-H, Lee E-J, Hung Y-C, Tai S-H, Chen H-Y, et al. Magnolol reduces glutamate-induced neuronal excitotoxicity and protects against permanent focal cerebral ischemia up to 4 hours. PLoS ONE. 2012;7(7):e39952.

45. Xiao X, Liu J, Hu J, Li T, Zhang Y. Protective effect of protopine on the focal cerebral ischaemic injury in rats. Basic Clin Pharmacol Toxicol. 2007;101(2):85–9.
46. Wang ZF, Wang J, Zhang HY, Tang XC. Huperzine a exhibits anti-inflammatory and neuroprotective effects in a rat model of transient focal cerebral ischemia. J Neurochem. 2008;106(4):1594–603.
47. Lee TH, Jung CH, Lee D-H. Neuroprotective effects of Schisandrin B against transient focal cerebral ischemia in Sprague-Dawley rats. Food Chem Toxicol. 2012;50(12):4239–45.
48. Thiyagarajan M, Sharma SS. Neuroprotective effect of curcumin in middle cerebral artery occlusion induced focal cerebral ischemia in rats. Life Sci. 2004;74(8):969–85.
49. Chen Y, Wu X, Yu S, Fauzee NJS, Wu J, Li L, et al. Neuroprotective capabilities of Tanshinone IIA against cerebral ischemia/reperfusion injury via anti-apoptotic pathway in rats. Biol Pharm Bull. 2012;35(2):164–70.
50. Ruan L, Huang H-S, Jin W-X, Chen H-M, Li X-J, Gong Q-J. Tetrandrine attenuated cerebral ischemia/reperfusion injury and induced differential proteomic changes in a MCAO mice model using 2-D DIGE. Neurochem Res. 2013;38(9):1871–9.
51. Zeng X, Zhang Y, Zhang S, Zheng X. A microdialysis study of effects of gastrodin on neurochemical changes in the ischemic/reperfused rat cerebral hippocampus. Biol Pharm Bull. 2007;30(4):801–4.
52. Egashira N, Hayakawa K, Osajima M, Mishima K, Iwasaki K, Oishi R, et al. Involvement of GABAA receptors in the neuroprotective effect of theanine on focal cerebral ischemia in mice. J Pharmacol Sci. 2007;105(2):211–4.
53. Kao T-K, Ou Y-C, J-s Kuo, Chen W-Y, Liao S-L, Wu C-W, et al. Neuroprotection by tetramethylpyrazine against ischemic brain injury in rats. Neurochem Int. 2006;48(3):166–76.
54. Zhang P, Liu X, Zhu Y, Chen S, Zhou D, Wang Y. Honokiol inhibits the inflammatory reaction during cerebral ischemia reperfusion by suppressing NF-κB activation and cytokine production of glial cells. Neurosci Lett. 2013;534:123–7.
55. Selkoe DJ. Cell biology of protein misfolding: the examples of Alzheimer's and Parkinson's diseases. Nature cell Biol. 2004;6(11):1054–61.
56. McKhann G, Drachman D, Folstein M, Katzman R, Price D, Stadlan EM. Clinical diagnosis of Alzheimer's disease: report of the NINCDS-ADRDA work group under the auspices of Department of Health and Human Services Task Force on Alzheimer's disease. Neurology. 1984;34(7):939–44.
57. Zarranz JJ, Alegre J, Gomez-Esteban JC, Lezcano E, Ros R, Ampuero I, et al. The new mutation, E46K, of alpha-synuclein causes Parkinson and Lewy body dementia. Ann Neurol. 2004;55(2):164–73.
58. Roth AD, Ramirez G, Alarcon R, Von Bernhardi R. Oligodendrocytes damage in Alzheimer's disease: beta amyloid toxicity and inflammation. Biol Res. 2005;38(4):381–7.
59. Oddo S, Caccamo A, Shepherd JD, Murphy MP, Golde TE, Kayed R, et al. Triple-transgenic model of Alzheimer's disease with plaques and tangles: intracellular A beta and synaptic dysfunction. Neuron. 2003;39(3):409–21.
60. Goedert M, Spillantini MG, Jakes R, Rutherford D, Crowther RA. Multiple isoforms of human microtubule-associated protein tau: sequences and localization in neurofibrillary tangles of Alzheimer's disease. Neuron. 1989;3(4):519–26.
61. Cheng TW, Chen TF, Yip PK, Hua MS, Yang CC, Chiu MJ. Comparison of behavioral and psychological symptoms of Alzheimer's disease among institution residents and memory clinic outpatients. Int Psychogeriatr. 2009;21(6):1134–41.
62. Dolan D, Troncoso J, Resnick SM, Crain BJ, Zonderman AB, O'Brien RJ. Age, Alzheimer's disease and dementia in the Baltimore longitudinal study of ageing. Brain J Neurol. 2010;133:2225–31.
63. Hirtz D, Thurman DJ, Gwinn-Hardy K, Mohamed M, Chaudhuri AR, Zalutsky R. How common are the "common" neurologic disorders? Neurology. 2007;68(5):326–37.
64. Alzheimer's A. Association Report. 2015 Alzheimer's disease facts and figures. Alzheimers Dement. 2015;11(3):332–84.

65. Games D, Adams D, Alessandrini R, Barbour R, Berthelette P, Blackwell C, et al. Alzheimer-type neuropathology in transgenic mice overexpressing V717F beta-amyloid precursor protein. Nature. 1995;373(6514):523–7.
66. Hsiao K, Chapman P, Nilsen S, Eckman C, Harigaya Y, Younkin S, et al. Correlative memory deficits, Abeta elevation, and amyloid plaques in transgenic mice. Science. 1996;274(5284):99–102.
67. Gotz J, Probst A, Spillantini MG, Schafer T, Jakes R, Burki K, et al. Somatodendritic localization and hyperphosphorylation of tau-protein in transgenic mice expressing the longest human brain tau-isoform. EMBO J. 1995;14(7):1304–13.
68. Chetelat G, Fouquet M. Neuroimaging biomarkers for Alzheimer's disease in asymptomatic APOE4 carriers. Rev Neurol France. 2013;169(10):729–36.
69. Raber J, Huang YD, Ashford JW. ApoE genotype accounts for the vast majority of AD risk and AD pathology. Neurobiol Aging. 2004;25(5):641–50.
70. Wang J, Tanila H, Puolivali J, Kadish I, van Groen T. Gender differences in the amount and deposition of amyloid beta in APPswe and PS1 double transgenic mice (vol. 14, p. 318, 2003). Neurobiol Dis. 2004;16(1):290.
71. Lewis J, Dickson DW, Lin WL, Chisholm L, Corral A, Jones G, et al. Enhanced neurofibrillary degeneration in transgenic mice expressing mutant tau and APP. Science. 2001;293(5534):1487–91.
72. Heraud C, Goufak D, Ando K, Leroy K, Suain V, Yilmaz Z, et al. Increased misfolding and truncation of tau in APP/PS1/tau transgenic mice compared to mutant tau mice. Neurobiol Dis. 2014;62:100–12.
73. WoodruffPak DS, Trojanowski JQ. The older rabbit as an animal model: implications for Alzheimer's disease. Neurobiol Aging. 1996;17(2):283–90.
74. Takeda T. Senescence-Accelerated Mouse (SAM) with special references to neurodegeneration models, SAMP8 and SAMP10 Mice. Neurochem Res. 2009;34(4):639–59.
75. Harkany T, O'Mahony S, Kelly JP, Soos K, Toro I, Penke B, et al. beta-Amyloid(Phe(SO3H)(24))25–35 in rat nucleus basalis induces behavioural dysfunctions, impairs learning and memory and disrupts cortical cholinergic innervation. Behav Brain Res. 1998;90(2):133–45.
76. Song XY, Hu JF, Chu SF, Zhang Z, Xu S, Yuan YH, et al. Ginsenoside Rg1 attenuates okadaic acid induced spatial memory impairment by the GSK3beta/tau signaling pathway and the Abeta formation prevention in rats. Eur J Pharmacol. 2013;710(1–3):29–38.
77. Raghavendra M, Maiti R, Kumar S, Acharya S. Role of aqueous extract of Azadirachta indica leaves in an experimental model of Alzheimer's disease in rats. Int J Appl Basic Med Res. 2013;3(1):37–47.
78. Lu MC. Danggui shaoyao san improve colchichine-induced learning acquisition impairment in rats. Acta Pharmacol Sin. 2001;22(12):1149–53.
79. Zhang Z, Yu CX. Effect of melatonin on learning and memory impairment induced by aluminum chloride and its mechanism. Yao xue xue bao (Acta Pharmaceutica Sinica). 2002;37(9):682–6.
80. Estape N, Steckler T. Cholinergic blockade impairs performance in operant DNMTP in two inbred strains of mice. Pharmacol Biochem Behav. 2002;72(1–2):319–34.
81. Luques L, Shoham S, Weinstock M. Chronic brain cytochrome oxidase inhibition selectively alters hippocampal cholinergic innervation and impairs memory: prevention by ladostigil. Exp Neurol. 2007;206(2):209–19.
82. Wang BS, Wang H, Wei ZH, Song YY, Zhang L, Chen HZ. Efficacy and safety of natural acetylcholinesterase inhibitor huperzine A in the treatment of Alzheimer's disease: an updated meta-analysis. J Neural Transm. 2009;116(4):457–65.
83. Ouyang S, Sun LS, Guo SL, Liu X, Xu JP. Effects of timosaponins on learning and memory abilities of rats with dementia induced by lateral cerebral ventricular injection of amyloid beta- peptide. Di 1 jun yi da xue xue bao (Academic Journal of the first medical college of PLA). 2005;25(2):121–6.

84. Leclerc S, Garnier M, Hoessel R, Marko D, Bibb JA, Snyder GL, et al. Indirubins inhibit glycogen synthase kinase-3 beta and CDK5/p25, two protein kinases involved in abnormal tau phosphorylation in Alzheimer's disease. A property common to most cyclin-dependent kinase inhibitors? J Biol Chem. 2001;276(1):251–60.
85. Weinmann S, Roll S, Schwarzbach C, Vauth C, Willich SN. Effects of Ginkgo biloba in dementia: systematic review and meta-analysis. BMC Geriatr. 2010;10.
86. Lu G, Wu Y, Mak YT, Wai SM, Feng ZT, Rudd JA, et al. Molecular evidence of the neuroprotective effect of Ginkgo biloba (EGb761) using bax/bcl-2 ratio after brain ischemia in senescence-accelerated mice, strain prone-8. Brain Res. 2006;1090:23–8.
87. Calapai G, Crupi A, Firenzuoli F, Marciano MC, Squadrito F, Inferrera G, et al. Neuroprotective effects of Ginkgo biloba extract in brain ischemia are mediated by inhibition of nitric oxide synthesis. Life Sci. 2000;67(22):2673–83.
88. Gauthier S, Schlaefke S. Efficacy and tolerability of Ginkgo biloba extract EGb 761 (R) in dementia: a systematic review and meta-analysis of randomized placebo-controlled trials. Clin Interv Aging. 2014;9:2065–77.
89. Wu JG, Wang YY, Zhang ZL, Yu B. Herbal medicine in the treatment of Alzheimer's disease. Chin J Integr Med. 2015;21(2):102–7.
90. Jia H, Jiang Y, Ruan Y, Zhang Y, Ma X, Zhang J, et al. Tenuigenin treatment decreases secretion of the Alzheimer's disease amyloid beta-protein in cultured cells. Neurosci Lett. 2004;367(1):123–8.
91. Asai M, Iwata N, Yoshikawa A, Aizaki Y, Ishiura S, Saido TC, et al. Berberine alters the processing of Alzheimer's amyloid precursor protein to decrease A beta secretion. Biochem Biophys Res Commun. 2007;352(2):498–502.
92. Wirths O, Multhaup G, Bayer TA. A modified beta-amyloid hypothesis: intraneuronal accumulation of the beta-amyloid peptide—the first step of a fatal cascade. J Neurochem. 2004;91(3):513–20.
93. Li Z, Li H, Zhao CH, Lv C, Zhong CJ, Xin WF, et al. Protective effect of Notoginsenoside R1 on an APP/PS1 mouse model of Alzheimer's disease by up-regulating insulin degrading enzyme and inhibiting A beta accumulation. Cns Neurol Disord. 2015;14(3):360–9.
94. Dauer W, Przedborski S. Parkinson's disease: mechanisms and models. Neuron. 2003;39 (6):889–909.
95. Chua CE, Tang BL. alpha-synuclein and Parkinson's disease: the first roadblock. J Cell Mol Med. 2006;10(4):837–46.
96. Blesa J, Trigo-Damas I, Quiroga-Varela A, Jackson-Lewis VR. Oxidative stress and Parkinson's disease. Front Neuroanat. 2015;9:91.
97. Hirsch EC, Hunot S, Damier P, Faucheux B. Glial cells and inflammation in Parkinson's disease: a role in neurodegeneration? Ann Neurol. 1998;44(3 Suppl 1):S115–20.
98. Nixon RA. The role of autophagy in neurodegenerative disease. Nature Med. 2013;19 (8):983–97.
99. Martin GE, Myers RD, Newberg DC. Catecholamine release by intracerebral perfusion of 6-hydroxydopamine and desipramine. Eur J Pharmacol. 1976;36(2):299–311.
100. Blandini F, Armentero MT, Martignoni E. The 6-hydroxydopamine model: news from the past. Parkinsonism Relat Disord. 2008;14(Suppl 2):S124–9.
101. Hacioglu G, Seval-Celik Y, Tanriover G, Ozsoy O, Saka-Topcuoglu E, Balkan S, et al. Docosahexaenoic acid provides protective mechanism in bilaterally MPTP-lesioned rat model of Parkinson's disease. Folia Histochem Cyto. 2012;50(2):228–38.
102. Inden M, Kitamura Y, Abe M, Tamaki A, Takata K, Taniguchi T. Parkinsonian rotenone mouse model: reevaluation of long-term administration of rotenone in C57BL/6 mice. Biol Pharm Bull. 2011;34(1):92–6.
103. Koller WC. Paraquat and Parkinson's disease. Neurology. 1986;36(8):1147.
104. Richfield EK, Thiruchelvam MJ, Cory-Slechta DA, Wuertzer C, Gainetdinov RR, Caron MG, et al. Behavioral and neurochemical effects of wild-type and mutated human alpha-synuclein in transgenic mice. Exp Neurol. 2002;175(1):35–48.

105. Masliah E, Rockenstein E, Veinbergs I, Mallory M, Hashimoto M, Takeda A, et al. Dopaminergic loss and inclusion body formation in alpha-synuclein mice: implications for neurodegenerative disorders. Science. 2000;287(5456):1265–9.
106. Rockenstein E, Mallory M, Hashimoto M, Song D, Shults CW, Lang I, et al. Differential neuropathological alterations in transgenic mice expressing alpha-synuclein from the platelet-derived growth factor and Thy-1 promoters. J Neurosci Res. 2002;68(5):568–78.
107. Gomez-Isla T, Irizarry MC, Mariash A, Cheung B, Soto O, Schrump S, et al. Motor dysfunction and gliosis with preserved dopaminergic markers in human alpha-synuclein A30P transgenic mice. Neurobiol Aging. 2003;24(2):245–58.
108. Zimprich A, Biskup S, Leitner P, Lichtner P, Farrer M, Lincoln S, et al. Mutations in LRRK2 cause autosomal-dominant parkinsonism with pleomorphic pathology. Neuron. 2004;44 (4):601–7.
109. Li XT, Patel JC, Wang J, Avshalumov MV, Nicholson C, Buxbaum JD, et al. Enhanced Striatal Dopamine transmission and motor performance with LRRK2 overexpression in mice is eliminated by familial Parkinson's disease mutation G2019S. J Neurosci. 2010;30 (5):1788–97.
110. Kumar A, Cookson MR. Role of LRRK2 kinase dysfunction in Parkinson disease. Expert Rev Mol Med. 2011;13.
111. Dawson TM, Ko HS, Dawson VL. Genetic animal models of Parkinson's disease. Neuron. 2010;66(5):646–61.
112. Kum WF, Durairajan SSK, Bian ZX, Man SC, Lam YC, Xie LX, et al. Treatment of Idiopathic Parkinson's disease with traditional chinese herbal medicine: a randomized placebo-controlled pilot clinical study. Evid Based Compl Alt. 2011:1–8.
113. Kim HG, Ju MS, Kim DH, Hong J, Cho SH, Cho KH, et al. Protective effects of Chunghyuldan against ROS-mediated neuronal cell death in models of Parkinson's disease. Basic Clin Pharmacol Toxicol. 2010;107(6):958–64.
114. Gao K, Liu MY, Cao JY, Yao MN, Lu YY, Li JK, et al. Protective effects of Lycium barbarum Polysaccharide on 6-OHDA-induced apoptosis in PC12 cells through the ROS-NO pathway. Molecules. 2015;20(1):293–308.
115. Li L, Yang N, Nin L, Zhao Z, Chen L, Yu J, et al. Chinese herbal medicine formula Tao Hong Si Wu Decoction protects against cerebral ischemia-reperfusion injury via PI3K/Akt and the Nrf2 signaling pathway. J Nat Med. 2015;69(1):76–85.
116. Ko C-N, Park I S, Park S-U, Jung W-S, Moon S-K, Park J-M, et al. Neuroprotective effect of Chunghyuldan (Qing Xue Dan) on hypoxia-reoxygenation induced damage of neuroblastoma 2a cell lines. Chin J Integr Med. 2013;19(12):940–4.
117. Li X-M, Bai X-C, Qin L-N, Huang H, Xiao Z-J, Gao T-M. Neuroprotective effects of Buyang Huanwu Decoction on neuronal injury in hippocampus after transient forebrain ischemia in rats. Neurosci Lett. 2003;346(1):29–32.
118. Lin Z, Zhu D, Yan Y, Yu B. Herbal formula FBD extracts prevented brain injury and inflammation induced by cerebral ischemia–reperfusion. J Ethnopharmacol. 2008;118 (1):140–7.
119. Wei X, Liu H, Sun X, Fu F, Zhang X, Wang J, et al. Hydroxysafflor yellow A protects rat brains against ischemia-reperfusion injury by antioxidant action. Neurosci Lett. 2005;386 (1):58–62.
120. Zhang GR, Cheng XR, Zhou WX, Zhang YX. Age-related expression of calcium/calmodulin-dependent protein kinase Ii a in the Hippocampus and cerebral cortex of senescence accelerated mouse prone/8 mice is modulated by anti-Alzheimer's disease drugs. Neuroscience. 2009;159(1):308–15.
121. Yang Y, Cheng XR, Zhang GR, Zhou WX, Zhang YX. Autocrine motility factor receptor is involved in the process of learning and memory in the central nervous system. Behav Brain Res. 2012;229(2):412–8.
122. Durairajan SS, Huang YY, Yuen PY, Chen LL, Kwok KY, Liu LF, et al. Effects of Huanglian-Jie-Du-Tang and its modified formula on the modulation of amyloid-beta precursor protein processing in Alzheimer's disease models. PLoS ONE. 2014;9(3):e92954.

123. Kim HG, Kim JY, Whang WW, Oh MS. Neuroprotective effect of Chunghyuldan from amyloid beta oligomer induced neuroinflammation in vitro and in vivo. Can J Physiol Pharm. 2014;92(6):429–37.
124. Wang L, Nishida H, Ogawa Y, Konishi T. Prevention of oxidative injury in PC12 cells by a traditional Chinese medicine, Shengmai San, as a model of an antioxidant-based composite formula. Biol Pharm Bull. 2003;26(7):1000–4.
125. Lin ZH, Xiao ZB, Zhu DN, Yan YQ, Yu BY, Wang QJ. Aqueous extracts of FBD, a Chinese herb formula composed of Poria cocos, Atractylodes macrocephala, and Angelica sinensis reverse scopolamine induced memory deficit in ICR mice. Pharm Biol. 2009;47(5):396–401.
126. Liu X, Hao WL, Qin YR, Decker Y, Wang X, Burkart M, et al. Long-term treatment with Ginkgo biloba extract EGb 761 improves symptoms and pathology in a transgenic mouse model of Alzheimer's disease. Brain Behav Immun. 2015;46:121–31.
127. Choi YT, Jung CH, Lee SR, Bae JH, Baek WK, Suh MH, et al. The green tea polyphenol (−)-epigallocatechin gallate attenuates beta-amyloid-induced neurotoxicity in cultured hippocampal neurons. Life Sci. 2001;70(5):603–14.
128. Guo J, Chang L, Zhang X, Pei S, Yu M, Gao J. Ginsenoside compound K promotes beta-amyloid peptide clearance in primary astrocytes via autophagy enhancement. Exp Ther Med. 2014;8(4):1271–4.
129. Xiao XQ, Wang R, Han YF, Tang XC. Protective effects of huperzine A on beta-amyloid (25–35) induced oxidative injury in rat pheochromocytoma cells. Neurosci Lett. 2000;286 (3):155–8.
130. Wang LM, Han YF, Tang XC. Huperzine A improves cognitive deficits caused by chronic cerebral hypoperfusion in rats. Eur J Pharmcol. 2000;398(1):65–72.
131. Yang L, Ye CY, Huang XT, Tang XC, Zhang HY. Decreased accumulation of subcellular amyloid-beta with improved mitochondrial function mediates the neuroprotective effect of huperzine A. J Alzheimer's Dis (JAD). 2012;31(1):131–42.
132. Zhang YH, Zhao XY, Chen XQ, Wang Y, Yang HH, Hu GY. Spermidine antagonizes the inhibitory effect of huperzine A on [3H]dizocilpine (MK-801) binding in synaptic membrane of rat cerebral cortex. Neurosci Lett. 2002;319(2):107–10.
133. Tang LL, Wang R, Tang XC. Effects of huperzine A on secretion of nerve growth factor in cultured rat cortical astrocytes and neurite outgrowth in rat PC12 cells. Acta Pharmacol Sin. 2005;26(6):673–8.
134. Yuan SM, Gao K, Wang DM, Quan XZ, Liu JN, Ma CM, et al. Evodiamine improves congnitive abilities in SAMP8 and APP(swe)/PS1(Delta E9) transgenic mouse models of Alzheimer's disease. Acta Pharmacol Sin. 2011;32(3):295–302.
135. Fan LH, Wang KZ, Cheng B, Wang CS, Dang XQ. Anti-apoptotic and neuroprotective effects of Tetramethylpyrazine following spinal cord ischemia in rabbits. BMC Neurosci. 2006;7:48.
136. Cheng XR, Zhang L, Hu JJ, Sun L, Du GH. Neuroprotective effects of tetramethylpyrazine on hydrogen peroxide-induced apoptosis in PC12 cells. Cell Biol Int. 2007;31(5):438–43.
137. Durairajan SS, Liu LF, Lu JH, Chen LL, Yuan Q, Chung SK, et al. Berberine ameliorates beta-amyloid pathology, gliosis, and cognitive impairment in an Alzheimer's disease transgenic mouse model. Neurobiol Aging. 2012;33(12):2903–19.
138. Xian YF, Lin ZX, Mao QQ, Hu Z, Zhao M, Che CT, et al. Bioassay-guided isolation of neuroprotective compounds from Uncaria rhynchophylla against Beta-Amyloid-induced neurotoxicity. Evid Based Complement Altern Med (eCAM). 2012;2012:802625.
139. Fujiwara H, Iwasaki K, Furukawa K, Seki T, He M, Maruyama M, et al. Uncaria rhynchophylla, a Chinese medicinal herb, has potent antiaggregation effects on Alzheimer's beta-amyloid proteins. J Neurosci Res. 2006;84(2):427–33.
140. Chen ZA, Wang JL, Liu RT, Ren JP, Wen LQ, Chen XJ, et al. Liquiritin potentiate neurite outgrowth induced by nerve growth factor in PC12 cells. Cytotechnology. 2009;60(1–3):125–32.

141. Ding HT, Wang HT, Zhao YX, Sun DK, Zhai X. Protective effects of Baicalin on A beta(1–42)-induced learning and memory deficit, oxidative stress, and apoptosis in rat. Cell Mol Neurobiol. 2015;35(5):623–32.
142. Yin F, Liu JH, Ji XH, Wang YW, Zidichouski J, Zhang JZ. Baicalin prevents the production of hydrogen peroxide and oxidative stress induced by A beta aggregation in SH-SY5Y cells. Neurosci Lett. 2011;492(2):76–9.
143. Xiong JX, Wang CZ, Chen HY, Hu YZ, Tian L, Pan JK, et al. A beta-induced microglial cell activation is inhibited by baicalin through the JAK2/STAT3 signaling pathway. Int J Neurosci. 2014;124(8):609–19.
144. Zeng KW, Ko H, Yang HO, Wang XM. Icariin attenuates beta-amyloid-induced neurotoxicity by inhibition of tau protein hyperphosphorylation in PC12 cells. Neuropharmacology. 2010;59(6):542–50.
145. Zhang H, Liu B, Wu J, Xu C, Tao J, Duan X, et al. Icariin inhibits corticosterone-induced apoptosis in hypothalamic neurons via the PI3K/Akt signaling pathway. Mol Med Rep. 2012;6(5):967–72.
146. Xing G, Dong M, Li X, Zou Y, Fan L, Wang X, et al. Neuroprotective effects of puerarin against beta-amyloid-induced neurotoxicity in PC12 cells via a PI3K-dependent signaling pathway. Brain Res Bull. 2011;85(3–4):212–8.
147. Wang HM, Wang LW, Liu XM, Li CL, Xu SP, Farooq AD. Neuroprotective effects of forsythiaside on learning and memory deficits in senescence-accelerated mouse prone (SAMP8) mice. Pharmacol Biochem Behav. 2013;105:134–41.
148. Dong X, Zhang D, Zhang L, Li W, Meng X. Osthole improves synaptic plasticity in the hippocampus and cognitive function of Alzheimer's disease rats via regulating glutamate. Neural Regeneration Res. 2012;7(30):2325–32.
149. Hu Y, Wen Q, Liang W, Kang T, Ren L, Zhang N, et al. Osthole reverses beta-amyloid peptide cytotoxicity on neural cells by enhancing cyclic AMP response element-binding protein phosphorylation. Biolo Pharm Bull. 2013;36(12):1950–8.
150. Tsai FS, Wu LY, Yang SE, Cheng HY, Tsai CC, Wu CR, et al. Ferulic acid reverses the cognitive dysfunction caused by amyloid beta peptide 1–40 through anti-oxidant activity and cholinergic activation in rats. Am J Chin Med. 2015;43(2):319–35.
151. Mao X, Liao Z, Guo L, Xu X, Wu B, Xu M, et al. Schisandrin C ameliorates learning and memory deficits by A beta -induced oxidative stress and neurotoxicity in mice. Phytotherapy Res PTR. 2015.
152. Huang JF, Shang L, Liu P, Zhang MQ, Chen S, Chen D, et al. Timosaponin-BII inhibits the up-regulation of BACE1 induced by Ferric Chloride in rat retina. BMC Complem Altern M. 2012;12.
153. Lv J, Jia H, Jiang Y, Ruan Y, Liu Z, Yue W, et al. Tenuifolin, an extract derived from tenuigenin, inhibits amyloid-beta secretion in vitro. Acta Physiol. 2009;196(4):419–25.
154. Hu YK, Li CY, Shen W. Gastrodin alleviates memory deficits and reduces neuropathology in a mouse model of Alzheimer's disease. Neuropathology. 2014;34(4):370–7.
155. Lv C, Wang L, Liu XL, Yan SJ, Yan SS, Wang YY, et al. Multi-faced neuroprotective effects of geniposide depending on the RAGE-mediated signaling in an Alzheimer mouse model. Neuropharmacology. 2015;89:175–84.
156. Wang Q, Xiao B, Cui SQ, Song HL, Qian YJ, Dong L, et al. Triptolide treatment reduces Alzheimer's disease (AD)-like pathology through inhibition of BACE1 in a transgenic mouse model of AD. Dis Model Mech. 2014;7(12):1385–95.
157. Wang C, Zhang X, Teng Z, Zhang T, Li Y. Downregulation of PI3K/Akt/mTOR signaling pathway in curcumin-induced autophagy in APP/PS1 double transgenic mice. Eur J Pharmacol. 2014;740:312–20.
158. Ju MS, Kim HG, Choi JG, Ryu JH, Hur J, Kim YJ, et al. Cassiae semen, a seed of Cassia obtusifolia, has neuroprotective effects in Parkinson's disease models. Food Chem Toxicol. 2010;48(8–9):2037–44.
159. Rojas P, Serrano-Garcia N, Mares-Samano JJ, Medina-Campos ON, Pedraza-Chaverri J, Ogren SO. EGb761 protects against nigrostriatal dopaminergic neurotoxicity in

1-methyl-4-phenyl-1,2,3,6-tetrahydropyridine-induced Parkinsonism in mice: role of oxidative stress. Eur J Neurosci. 2008;28(1):41–50.
160. Kim EH, Jang MH, Shin MC, Shin MS, Kim CJ. Protective effect of aqueous extract of Ginseng radix against 1-methyl-4-phenylpyridinium-induced apoptosis in PC12 cells. Biol Pharm Bull. 2003;26(12):1668–73.
161. Lu JH, Tan JQ, Durairajan SSK, Liu LF, Zhang ZH, Ma L, et al. Isorhynchophylline, a natural alkaloid, promotes the degradation of alpha-synuclein in neuronal cells via inducing autophagy (vol. 8, p. 98, 2012). Autophagy. 2012;8(5):864–6.
162. Chen LL, Song JX, Lu JH, Yuan ZW, Liu LF, Durairajan SSK, et al. Corynoxine, a natural autophagy enhancer, promotes the clearance of Alpha-Synuclein via Akt/mTOR pathway. J Neuroimmune Pharm. 2014;9(3):380–7.
163. Zhang X, Xiong J, Liu S, Wang L, Huang J, Liu L, et al. Puerarin protects dopaminergic neurons in Parkinson's disease models. Neuroscience. 2014;280:88–98.
164. Sheng GQ, Pu XP, Lei L, Tu PF, Li CL. Tubuloside B from Cistanche salsa rescues the PC12 neuronal cells from 1-methyl-4-phenylpyridinium ion-induced apoptosis and oxidative stress. Planta Med. 2002;68(11):966–70.
165. Geng XC, Song LW, Pu XP, Tu PF. Neuroprotective effects of phenylethanoid glycosides from Cistanches salsa against 1-methyl-4-phenyl-1,2,3,6-tetrahydropyridine (MPTP) induced dopaminergic toxicity in C57 mice. Biol Pharm Bull. 2004;27(6):797–801.
166. Hwang YP, Jeong HG. Ginsenoside Rb1 protects against 6-hydroxydopamine-induced oxidative stress by increasing heme oxygenase-1 expression through an estrogen receptor-related PI3 K/Akt/Nrf2-dependent pathway in human dopaminergic cells. Toxicol Appl Pharmacol. 2010;242(1):18–28.
167. Radad K, Gille G, Moldzio R, Saito H, Ishige K, Rausch WD. Ginsenosides Rb1 and Rg1 effects on survival and neurite growth of MPP+ -affected mesencephalic dopaminergic cells. J Neural Transm. 2004;111(1):37–45.
168. Xu BB, Liu CQ, Gao X, Zhang WQ, Wang SW, Cao YL. Possible mechanisms of the protection of ginsenoside Re against MPTP-induced apoptosis in substantia nigra neurons of Parkinson's disease mouse model. J Asian Nat Prod Res. 2005;7(3):215–24.
169. Tian LL, Wang XJ, Sun YN, Li CR, Xing YL, Zhao HB, et al. Salvianolic acid B, an antioxidant from Salvia miltiorrhiza, prevents 6-hydroxydopamine induced apoptosis in SH-SY5Y cells. Int J Biochem Cell B. 2008;40(3):409–22.
170. Wang SX, Jing HR, Yang HY, Liu ZD, Guo H, Chai LJ, et al. Tanshinone I selectively suppresses pro-inflammatory genes expression in activated microglia and prevents nigrostriatal dopaminergic neurodegeneration in a mouse model of Parkinson's disease. J Ethnopharm. 2015;164:247–55.
171. Xue X, Liu H, Qi L, Li X, Guo C, Gong D, et al. Baicalein ameliorated the upregulation of striatal glutamatergic transmission in the mice model of Parkinson's disease. Brain Res Bull. 2014;103:54–9.
172. Lee E, Park HR, Ji ST, Lee Y, Lee J. Baicalein attenuates astroglial activation in the 1-methyl-4-phenyl-1,2,3,4-tetrahydropyridine-induced Parkinson's disease model by downregulating the activations of nuclear factor-kappaB, ERK, and JNK. J Neurosci Res. 2014;92(1):130–9.
173. Lu JH, Ardah MT, Durairajan SSK, Liu LF, Xie LX, Fong WFD, et al. Baicalein inhibits formation of alpha-Synuclein Oligomers within living cells and prevents A beta peptide fibrillation and oligomerisation. ChemBioChem. 2011;12(4):615–24.
174. Xiong P, Chen X, Guo C, Zhang N, Ma B. Baicalin and deferoxamine alleviate iron accumulation in different brain regions of Parkinson's disease rats. Neural Regeneration Res. 2012;7(27):2092–8.
175. Guo CY, Chen X, Xiong P. Baicalin suppresses iron accumulation after substantia nigra injury: relationship between iron concentration and transferrin expression. Neural Regeneration Res. 2014;9(6):630–6.

176. Li LY, Zhao XL, Fei XF, Gu ZL, Qin ZH, Liang ZQ. Bilobalide inhibits 6-OHDA-induced activation of NF-kappaB and loss of dopaminergic neurons in rat substantia nigra. Acta Pharmacol Sin. 2008;29(5):539–47.
177. Kim M, Cho KH, Shin MS, Lee JM, Cho HS, Kim CJ, et al. Berberine prevents nigrostriatal dopaminergic neuronal loss and suppresses hippocampal apoptosis in mice with Parkinson's disease. Int J Mol Med. 2014;33(4):870–8.
178. Zhao H, Xu ML, Zhang Q, Guo ZH, Peng Y, Qu ZY, et al. Tetramethylpyrazine alleviated cytokine synthesis and dopamine deficit and improved motor dysfunction in the mice model of Parkinson's disease. Neurol Sci. 2014;35(12):1963–7.
179. Magalingam KB, Radhakrishnan A, Ramdas P, Haleagrahara N. Quercetin glycosides induced neuroprotection by changes in the gene expression in a cellular model of Parkinson's disease. J Mol Neurosci. 2015;55(3):609–17.
180. Ahsan N, Mishra S, Jain MK, Surolia A, Gupta S. Curcumin Pyrazole and its derivative (N-(3-nitrophenylpyrazole) curcumin inhibit aggregation, disrupt fibrils and modulate toxicity of wild type and mutant alpha-Synuclein. Sci Rep. 2015;5:9862.
181. Ji HF, Shen L. The multiple pharmaceutical potential of curcumin in Parkinson's disease. Cns Neurol Disord. 2014;13(2):369–73.
182. Zhang LB, Liu XH, Jiang Y, Guo P, Sha LJ, Li Y. Effect of notoginsenoside-Rg(1) on the expression of several proteins in the striatum of rat models with Parkinson's disease. Chem Res Chin U. 2006;22(2):139–44.
183. Lofrumento DD, Nicolardi G, Cianciulli A, De Nuccio F, La Pesa V, Carofiglio V, et al. Neuroprotective effects of resveratrol in an MPTP mouse model of Parkinson's-like disease: possible role of SOCS-1 in reducing pro-inflammatory responses. Innate Immun London. 2014;20(3):249–60.
184. Ferretta A, Gaballo A, Tanzarella P, Piccoli C, Capitanio N, Nico B, et al. Effect of resveratrol on mitochondrial function: Implications in parkin-associated familiar Parkinson's disease. Bba-Mol Basis Dis. 2014;1842(7):902–15.

Chapter 11
Effects of Chinese Medicinal Components on Chemokine Receptors: Theory, Results, and Methodology

Jiang He, Zhen-dan He and Xin Chen

Abstract Chemokine receptors are involved in a broad spectrum of physiological and pathological processes that include immune responses, inflammation, viral infection, as well as development and metastasis of cancer. Targeting of chemokine receptors has become a therapeutic strategy and the selective chemokine receptor antagonists have important therapeutic implications. One of such examples is the anti-HIV effect of inhibitors of CC-chemokine receptor 5 (CCR5) and CXC chemokine receptor 4 (CXCR4). Chinese medicines (CM) have been used for the treatment of inflammatory diseases for thousands of years, however, the scientific basis for the beneficial clinical effects of CM remains to be fully understood. So far, our studies have identified a number of chemokine receptor antagonists with defined chemical structures from CM with anti-inflammatory properties. These naturally occurring compounds have in vitro activity in the blockade of binding of chemokine ligands to their receptors, and consequently inhibited the chemotactic migration of leukocytes induced by certain chemokines. Our studies indicate that the clinical efficacy of anti-inflammatory CM is at least partially attributable to their inhibitory effect on chemokine receptors. Therefore, identification of CM-derived compounds capable of targeting chemokine receptors can unveil mechanisms underlying the anti-inflammatory effect of CM, and may also lead to the development of novel therapeutic agents. This chapter summarizes and discusses some of the recent studies in this field and the relevant experimental protocols are also introduced.

J. He · X. Chen (✉)
State Key Laboratory of Quality Research in Chinese Medicine, Institute of Chinese Medical Sciences, University of Macau, Macau, China
e-mail: xchen@umac.mo

J. He
e-mail: mb55825@umac.mo

Z. He
Department of Pharmacy, School of Medicine, Shenzhen University, Shenzhen 518060, China
e-mail: hezhendan@szu.edu.cn

S. Leung and H. Hu (eds.), *Evidence-based Research Methods for Chinese Medicine*, DOI 10.1007/978-981-10-2290-6_11

Keywords Chemokine · Chemokine receptor · Antagonist · Chinese medicines

11.1 Introduction

Chemokines are a family of chemotactic cytokines that direct the migration and positioning of certain cell subsets. According to the site of the first two cysteines that is adjacent to the amino terminus, chemokines have been classified into four highly conserved groups—CXC, CC, C, and CX3C [1]. By targeting their receptors, chemokines and chemokine receptors have pivotal roles in inflammation, homeostasis, and metastasis. So far, up to 50 endogenous chemokine ligands and 20 signaling chemokine receptors have been identified. These receptors are G protein-coupled receptors (GPCRs) that constitute the largest branch of the γ subfamily of rhodopsin-like seven transmembrane receptors [2]. It has been shown that the dysregulation of chemokine system involves in the inflammatory diseases [such as atherosclerosis, pulmonary disease, multiple sclerosis (MS), rheumatoid arthritis (RA), psoriasis, atopic dermatitis, and inflammatory bowel disease (IBD)], the infectious disease (HIV infection), cancer, and stem cell mobilization [3]. Thus, small molecule inhibitors of chemokine receptors have been intensively pursued as therapeutic agents by pharmaceutical companies as well as research institutes. To date, two of such compounds have been approved for the treatment of specific diseases: Maraviroc, targeting CC-chemokine receptor 5 (CCR5), and AMD 3100, targeting CXC chemokine receptor 4 (CXCR4) [4, 5]. There were several failed Phase II clinical studies, and none compound has been approved for the treatment of inflammatory and/or autoimmune diseases.

Chinese medicines (CM) have been used in the prescriptions for chronic inflammatory diseases, including RA, allergic asthma, liver injury and genital infection historically [6–10]. Some studies suggest that the anti-inflammatory effect of CM is on the basis of the inhibition of chemokines' biological activity or blockade of chemokine receptors' functions [11]. Therefore, further study may yield novel compounds from CM with the capacity to potently inhibit chemokine receptors' functions. Such compounds may merit future research and development into novel anti-inflammatory agents.

GPCR appears to be a "superstar" in the new drug research and development. In the United States, more than 30 % of all marketed therapeutics target on these proteins [12]. Unlike other cytokines with pleiotropic effects, chemokines only act on specific subsets of cells such as leukocytes to induce migration of these cells even without activating them in some cases. In this regard, blockade of a chemokine or its receptor may have a relatively specific effect, therefore endowing them with minimal adverse effects. Nevertheless, efforts in the development of novel and effective chemokine receptor antagonists were quite frustrating. Several promising compounds failed to enter into Phase III trials. These compounds were developed by companies including Millennium (CCR1 and CCR2 antagonists), Merck (CCR2 antagonist), Berlex/Schering (CCR1 antagonist), and Amgen/Tularik (CXCR3 antagonist). The halt of trials was mainly due to a lack of efficacy [4]. It was probably caused by a number of reasons [4, 5, 13]. For example, the levels of drug in the plasma were insufficient to neutralize the activity of the receptors. Some of small molecule inhibitors had off-target effects; or owned poor drug-like properties. And some of those antagonists had effect on experimental animals, but not on human subjects, due to the differences of the immune systems between human beings and animals. Furthermore, the redundancy of chemokine receptor function also mitigated the effect of specific inhibitor.

Screening compounds from CM for chemokine receptor antagonists has some advantages. Unlike the standard procedures of developing a new drug, CM have been employed in the treatment of human diseases for centuries and the efficacy has been firmly established. Further, recent laboratory research provided wealth scientific evidences of CM. Therefore, components identified from CM with the capacity of blocking chemokine receptors are likely to be active in human patients. Furthermore, studies show that some compounds from CM targeted several chemokine receptors simultaneously [14]. This property may be exploited to overcome the redundancy of functions of chemokine receptors.

This chapter provides a new insight into the theory of developing small molecule chemokine receptor antagonists from CM. Evidence and mechanism of Chinese herb-derived components with the capacity of directly targeting chemokine receptors will be discussed. Methodology of the relevant studies will also be introduced.

11.2 Inhibitory Effects of CM Components on Chemokine Receptors

CM are widely used in China and other Asian countries in the treatment of various inflammatory diseases including RA. Their clinical efficacy is partially based on the capacity of targeting GPCRs, as shown by recent laboratory research [15]. And a considerable effort has been made by researchers to pursue small-molecule antagonists of GPCRs with good bioavailability from CM [16]. It has also been shown the extract of CM used for the treatment of arthritis inhibited the migration of mast cells, presumably by interfering the interaction of chemokine and its receptor [17]. Our group has identified a number of chemokine/chemokine receptor inhibitors from CM with anti-inflammatory effects. Although modulation of the expression of pro-inflammatory cytokines and chemokines/chemokine receptors is likely to be one of major effect of anti-inflammatory CM [18], it is not included in this review.

11.2.1 Shikonin

Shikonin isolated from the Chinese herbal medicine *Zicao* (dried roots of *Lithospermum erythrorhizon*) is a naphthoquinone pigment that shows potent anti-inflammatory capacity [19]. It has been used in the treatment of inflammatory or autoimmune diseases, including RA, IBD, asthma, lupus nephritis, acute pancreatitis (AP), and lung injury, and its anti-inflammatory effect has also been shown in some in vivo models [20–26]. Moreover, the derivatives of shikonin have effects of inhibiting complete Freunds adjuvant-induced chronic arthritis in rats [27]. In a previous study, our group found that shikonin blocked regulated upon activation, normal T-cell expressed, and secreted (RANTES or CCL5) and macrophage inflammatory protein-1α (MIP-1α or CCL3) binding to CCR1 and thus inhibited RANTES other than epidermal growth factor (EGF)-induced migration of human embryonic kidney (HEK) cells [28]. Furthermore, our investigation also showed that shikonin, at nanomolar concentration, inhibited monocyte chemotaxis and calcium flux in response to a broad spectrum of CC chemokines (monocyte-chemoattractant protein-1, MCP-1, or CCL2, MIP-1α/CCL3, and RANTES/CCL5), CXC chemokine (stromal cell-derived factor-1α, SDF-1α or CXCL12), and classic chemoattractants (*N*-Formylmethionyl-leucyl-phenylalanine, fMLP and complement fraction C5a). Blockade of signaling pathways of these receptors was speculated to be responsible for the effects. Surface expression of CCR5, a primary HIV-1 co-receptor, on macrophages to a greater degree than the other receptors (CCR1, CCR2, CXCR4, and the formyl peptide receptor, FPR) as well as mRNA levels was down-regulated by shikonin simultaneously. Furthermore, shikonin inhibited the replication of a multidrug-resistant strain and pediatric clinical isolates of HIV in human peripheral blood mononuclear cells. Our results suggest that the anti-HIV and anti-inflammatory activities of shikonin may be related to its inhibition of the expression and function of chemokine receptors [14]. Moreover, as aforementioned, multiple-receptor antagonist is a possible way to overcome the hurdle of redundancy of the targets, for example, several chemokine receptors are associated with the pathogenesis of RA. Thus, as a pan chemokine receptor inhibitor, shikonin can be a promising candidate for developing novel anti-arthritic or other anti-inflammatory chemokine receptor antagonist.

11.2.2 Bile Acid

Niuhuang (termed as calculus bovis, bezaor bovin, or ox gallstone), a biliary product supposed to be able to remove heat and toxic substances in CM theory, has showed immunosuppressive effect in previous report [29]. Bile acids (deoxycholic acid, DCA, and cholic acid, CA) are major bioactive compounds of CM contain *Niuhuang* or other kinds of biliary products. *Qing Kai Ling* (QKL), a multicomponent herbal injection contains *Niuhuang-derived* DCA, was reported to inhibit a number of chemokine and classic chemoattractant-induced leukocyte migration, including blockade of fMLP-induced leukocyte migration by our group [30]. Consequently, we observed that fMLP-induced chemotaxis and calcium mobilization of monocyte and neutrophil were inhibited by DCA markedly. The binding of [^{3}H]fMLP and anti-FPR monoclonal antibodies (mAb) to the cells was also blocked by DCA. The inhibitory effects of DCA on calcium mobilization and anti-FPR-mAb binding to the receptor could be abrogated by washing DCA out of the cell suspension, suggesting that DCA blocked fMLP receptors via a steric hindrance mechanism, not via receptor internalization. However, DCA had no significant inhibitory effects on MCP-1, SDF-1α, or C5a-induced monocyte function, or C5a- or interleukin (IL)-8-induced neutrophil function. These results suggested that blockade of fMLP receptors might contribute to the anti-inflammatory effects of CM containing DCA [30]. Moreover, chenodeoxycholic acid (CDCA) and ursodeoxycholic acid (UDCA), two derivatives of DCA also showed inhibitory effects on FPR and FPR-like-1 (FPRL1), though less potent than DCA [31]. Since therapeutically targeting of FPRL1 inhibits inflammation in patients with arthritis [32], this activity of bile acids (DCA, CDCA, and UDCA) is likely to contribute to their effect in the treatment of RA [33–35].

11.2.3 Tannic Acid

We also found that *Shuang Huang Lian* injection (SHHL, an injectable multiple CM preparation) inhibited certain chemokine-induced chemotaxis previously. By testing the activity of fractions from the aqueous extracts of SHHL ingredients, we found that an extract of *Lianqiao* (dried fruit of *Forsythia suspense*) potently inhibited radiolabeled SDF-1α binding to cells. Guided by binding assay, we sequentially purified active compounds in extract of *Lianqiao* by chromatography procedures and found that a tannic acid was able to block SDF-1α receptors. Tannic acid, at nontoxic concentrations (IC_{50}, 7.5 μg/ml), specifically inhibited SDF-1α/CXCL12-induced human monocyte migration but did not inhibit MCP-1/CCL2, MIP-1α/CCL3, RANTES/CCL5, fMLP, or C5a-induced cell migration. It markedly blocked SDF-1α/CXCL12 binding to THP-1 (a human leukemia monocytic cell line) cells (IC_{50}, 0.36 μg/ml). Tannic acid also inhibited SDF-1α/CXCL12-induced, but not EGF-induced, migration of MDA 231 breast tumor cells. In addition, tannic acid (0.5 μg/ml) selectively inhibited SDF-1α/CXCL12-mediated, but not basic fibroblast growth factor (bFGF)- or endothelial cell growth supplement-mediated, bovine aorta endothelial cell (BAEC) capillary tube formation [36]. In this case, tannic acid not only inhibited chemotaxis but also angiogenesis induced by the interaction of SDF-1α/CXCR4. Furthermore, SDF-1α/CXCR4 axis is pivotal in retention of inflammatory cells in the synovium and angiogenesis in RA [37, 38] and blockade of SDF-1α/CXCR4 interaction by different agents has shown beneficial effect [39, 40]. Tannic acid has been reported to inhibit adjuvant-induced polyarthritis in rat and to inhibit leukocyte migration to the inflammatory site [41]. Therefore, blockade of SDF-1α/CXCR4 interaction may be one mechanism underlying the anti-arthritic effect of tannic acid. Since tannic acid is abundant in the plant kingdom, the impact of tannic acid in the daily dietary vegetables and grains on the RA is merit for further study.

11.3 Methodology

Chemokines act largely on leukocytes and have been shown to induce the directional (chemotactic) and random (chemokinetic) migration of selected cell types including neutrophils, monocytes, lymphocytes, eosinophils, basophils, mast cells, and fibroblasts. Some of these cytokines have also been shown to induce respiratory burst, enzyme release, degranulation, intracellular free Ca^{2+} mobilization, cellular polarization, morphologic changes, actin polymerization, and an increase in adherence of leukocytes to endothelium and extracellular matrix. Each of the major subclasses of chemokines has been shown to be selective for a particular subset of leukocytes [42]. Though leukocyte degranulation assay, pH changes assay, respiratory burst assay, actin polymerization assay, cellular polarization assay, and cell adhesion assay can be employed in the experiments, in this review, we focus on the introduction of major methods for the research on the inhibitory effect of CM on chemokine receptor functions [42, 43].

11.3.1 Chemotaxis Assay

Chemotaxis assay is a sensitive method to evaluate the capacity of cell migration while easy to perform. Thus, the primary screening of chemokine receptor antagonists from CM can be performed at most laboratories. It is similar to assess monocyte chemotaxis and granulocyte chemotaxis, however monocytes and dendritic cells are permitted to migrate in response to a chemokine gradient across a polyvinylpyrrolidone (PVP)-coated polycarbonate filter [42]. Nitrocellulose filters can also be used for chemotaxis assay with the advantage of quantifying the relatively accurate distance that a cell traffics in response to any given chemokine. Meanwhile, fluorescence-based assay provides a rapid qualitative measurement of cell migration, and requires fewer cells per well and permits the examination of more groups per chamber.

The protocol of chemotaxis assay is briefly introduced as following. Appropriately diluted chemokines or chemoattractants are loaded into the wells in the lower compartment. Cell suspension is placed in the upper compartment of the well. A polycarbonate filter is used to separate these two compartments. CM or CM-derived compounds, diluted with chemotaxis medium, can be added to the chemokine/chemoattractant, or added to the cells, depending on the purpose of experiments. After incubation for certain time according to the cell type, the filter is removed, fixed, and stained with DiffQuik. The cells on the underside of the membrane are counted at a 200× magnification microscopy. And data can be expressed as absolute number of cells migrated or as chemotactic index (CI), which represents the fold increase in the number of cells migrate in response to chemoattractants over the cell response to control medium [30].

11.3.2 Calcium Mobilization

Binding of chemokines to their receptors also results in the elevation of cytosolic calcium as an early biochemical event in leukocytes. Intracellular free calcium is usually maintained at low levels by a calcium gradient through ion pumps and by association of calcium into various intracellular compartments and cell membranes. Chemokine receptor activation normally leads to the release of membrane-associated calcium through the release of inositol triphosphate (IP3) and phospholipases. IP3 subsequently induces the release of calcium from endoplasmic reticulum, which in turn leads to an opening of the calcium channels on the plasma membrane and the additional influx of extracellular calcium. The development of fluorescent dyes that are trapped intracellular enables the monitoring of the cytosolic calcium concentration. Calcium mobilization is typically measured using acetoxymethyl (AM) esters of fluorescent dyes such as indo-1 and fura-2, two fluorescent calcium dyes that undergo a change in fluorescent properties upon binding free calcium. The emission ratio dye indo-1 exhibits a change in emission spectrum upon binding calcium and the ratio of bound fluorescence to unbound is used to estimate the calcium concentration [42]. Chemokine-induced calcium flux can also be detected by flow cytometry [44], and different methods to load indo-1 or fura-2 into cells have been developed for the experiments [45].

Following is a brief introduction of the procedure of conventional calcium mobilization assay. Monocytes, neutrophils, or other cells are incubated in loading buffer with Fura-2. The Fura-2-loaded cells are washed and resuspended in fresh loading buffer and then transferred into quartz cuvettes that are placed in a luminescence spectrometer LS50 B. Chemokines and CM compounds at different concentrations are added to the cuvettes at indicated time points. Results are acquired from the ratio of fluorescence at 340 and 380 nm wavelengths that is calculated by the FL WinLab (Perkin Elmer) program [46].

11.3.3 Binding Assay

To further verify the effect of chemokine receptor antagonist, the ligand binding experiments can be employed with the radiolabeled chemokine ligand. Briefly, a specific concentration of radiolabeled chemokine ligand is incubated with human leukocyte or cell line transfected with chemoattractant receptor in the presence of increasing concentrations of unlabeled chemokines, or in the presence of different concentration of CM or CM-derived compounds. The protocol is also briefly introduced as following. Cells are washed once with ice-cold PBS then are layered onto a 10 % sucrose/PBS cushion in Eppendorf tubes after incubation. The cells are centrifuged and the tips of the tubes containing cell pellets are cut and measured for radioactivity using a gamma counter. The binding data can be analyzed and plotted with a computer-aided program LIGAND (P. Munson, Division of Computer

Research and Technology, NIH, Bethesda, MD). The level of specific binding is determined by subtraction of nonspecific binding (cpm on cells in the presence of 1 μM unlabeled chemokines) from the total binding (cpm on cells in the absence of unlabeled chemokines) [46].

Radiolabeled ligands has remained the gold-standard method in binding assay, however, fluorescence-based techniques have also been developed as an alternative method. For example, flow cytometric technique can employ commercially available fluorescent chemokine ligand as a probe in binding assay. Alexa Fluor 647 conjugate of CXCL12 was used to test the effect of AMD3100, a well-known CXCR4 inhibitor [47]. It was reported a nonradioactive binding assay, using fluorescence-based technology named Tag-lite®, was applicable in high-throughput screening (HTS) [48]. Thus, those less harzardous nonradioactive binding assay can also be applicable in the study of TCM-derived inhibitors of chemokine receptors.

11.3.4 FITC-Bearing Dendritic Cells Migration Assay

Our group has employed an in vivo migration assay for dendritic cells, a method previously reported by Fukunaga et al. [49]. Briefly, FITC is first dissolved in acetone/dibutylphthalate in a ratio of 1:1 before usage. Mice are then painted on the halves of the dorsal ear with 10 μL of 1 % FITC solution. Mice are pretreated with CM extracts. Draining auricular lymph nodes are collected 24 h after FITC painting and then placed in RPMI 1640 medium. After that single cell suspension is prepared and the cell number determined. Then the cells are incubated on ice for 30 min with PE-conjugated anti-mouse CD11c mAbs or isotype control, respectively. The number and proportion of FITC-expressing $CD11^+$ cells, for example, dendritic cells migrated from skin to the draining lymphoid nodes can be analyzed by this method [50].

11.4 Concluding Remarks

Extensive studies have aimed to develop small molecule inhibitors for chemokine receptors that could overcome current hurdles in the treatment of inflammation and autoimmune diseases. Efforts have also been made to unveil the mechanisms of anti-inflammatory effects of CM from the aspect of acting on chemokine receptors, resulting in the identification of shikonin, bile acid, and tannic acid as antagonists of chemokine receptor. These compounds represent major active components of three CM products which have been used for centuries in the treatment of inflammatory diseases. Therefore, inhibition of chemokine receptor function should attribute, at least partially, to the clinical efficacy of some anti-inflammatory CM products. Further study may lead to the discovery of more potent small-molecule antagonists of chemokine receptors from CM, which may be able to develop into therapeutic agents. The methodology introduced in this review, such as chemotaxis assay, calcium mobilization assay and binding assay, could be employed by the investigators in their studies aiming at discovery of novel chemokine receptor inhibitors from CM.

Acknowledgments This study was supported by the Macao Science and Technology Development Fund (011/2015/A), and a grant from the University of Macau (Project No. MYRG2014-00024-ICMS-QRCM).

References

1. Murphy PM, Baggiolini M, Charo IF, Hebert CA, Horuk R, Matsushima K, et al. International union of pharmacology. XXII. Nomenclature for chemokine receptors. Pharmacol Rev. 2000;52(1):145–76. (PubMed PMID: 10699158).
2. Griffith JW, Sokol CL, Luster AD. Chemokines and chemokine receptors: positioning cells for host defense and immunity. Annu Rev Immunol. 2014;32:659–702.
3. Garin A, Proudfoot AE. Chemokines as targets for therapy. Exp Cell Res. 2011;317(5):602–12.
4. Horuk R. Chemokine receptor antagonists: overcoming developmental hurdles. Nat Rev Drug Discov. 2009;8(1):23–33. (PubMed PMID: 19079127).
5. Schall TJ, Proudfoot AE. Overcoming hurdles in developing successful drugs targeting chemokine receptors. Nat Rev Immunol. 2011;11(5):355–63. (PubMed PMID: 21494268).
6. Cyong J, Otsuka Y. A pharmacological study of the anti-inflammatory activity of Chinese herbs. A review. Acupunct Electrother Res. 1982;7(2–3):173–202. (PubMed PMID: 6128873).
7. Ho LJ, Lai JH. Chinese herbs as immunomodulators and potential disease-modifying antirheumatic drugs in autoimmune disorders. Curr Drug Metab. 2004;5(2):181–92. (PubMed PMID: 15078195).
8. Zhang T, Srivastava K, Wen MC, Yang N, Cao J, Busse P, et al. Pharmacology and immunological actions of a herbal medicine ASHMI on allergic asthma. Phytother Res. 2010;24(7):1047–55. (PubMed PMID: 19998324).
9. Liu C, Zhang Y, Kong S, Tsui I, Yu Y, Han F. Applications and therapeutic actions of complementary and alternative medicine for women with genital infection. Evid Based Complement Alternat Med. 2014;2014:658624. (PubMed PMID: 24648850. Pubmed Central PMCID: 3932255).
10. He J, Hu XP, Zeng Y, Li Y, Wu HQ, Qiu RZ, et al. Advanced research on acteoside for chemistry and bioactivities. J Asian Nat Prod Res. 2011;13(5):449–64. (PubMed PMID: 21534045).
11. Chen X, Oppenheim JJ, Howard OM. Chemokines and chemokine receptors as novel therapeutic targets in rheumatoid arthritis (RA): inhibitory effects of traditional Chinese medicinal components. Cell Mol Immunol. 2004;1(5):336–42. (PubMed PMID: 16285892).
12. Hopkins AL, Groom CR. The druggable genome. Nat Rev Drug Discov. 2002;1(9):727–30. (PubMed PMID: 12209152.)
13. Therapeutic targeting of chemokine receptors by small molecules. Drug Discov Today Technol. 2012;9(4):e227–314. (PubMed PMID: 24063737).
14. Chen X, Yang L, Zhang N, Turpin JA, Buckheit RW, Osterling C, et al. Shikonin, a component of chinese herbal medicine, inhibits chemokine receptor function and suppresses human immunodeficiency virus type 1. Antimicrob Agents Chemother. 2003;47(9):2810-6. (PubMed PMID: 12936978. Pubmed Central PMCID: 182643).

15. Im DS. Linking Chinese medicine and G-protein-coupled receptors. Trends Pharmacol Sci. 2003;24(1):2–4. (PubMed PMID: 12498721).
16. Horuk R. Development and evaluation of pharmacological agents targeting chemokine receptors. Methods. 2003;29(4):369–75. (PubMed PMID: 12725804).
17. Kim MS, Choi IY, Lee SH, Hong SH, Shin T, Kim HM. The Oriental medicine "Cool-Cool (Cool-X-A)" inhibits inflammatory cytokine production and migration in mast cells. Biol Pharm Bull. 2004;27(1):34–7. (PubMed PMID: 14709895).
18. Chen X, Krakauer T, Oppenheim JJ, Howard OM. Yin zi huang, an injectable multicomponent chinese herbal medicine, is a potent inhibitor of T-cell activation. J Altern Complement Med. 2004;10(3):519–26. (PubMed PMID: 15253857).
19. Chen X, Yang L, Oppenheim JJ, Howard MZ. Cellular pharmacology studies of shikonin derivatives. Phytother Res. 2002;16(3):199–209. (PubMed PMID: 12164262).
20. Andujar I, Rios JL, Giner RM, Recio MC. Pharmacological properties of shikonin—a review of literature since 2002. Planta Med. 2013;79(18):1685–97. (PubMed PMID: 24155261).
21. Bai GZ, Yu HT, Ni YF, Li XF, Zhang ZP, Su K, et al. Shikonin attenuates lipopolysaccharide-induced acute lung injury in mice. J Surg Res. 2013;182(2):303–11. (PubMed PMID: 23158409).
22. Dai Q, Fang J, Zhang FS. Dual role of shikonin in early and late stages of collagen type II arthritis. Mol Biol Rep. 2009;36(6):1597–604. (PubMed PMID: 18781399).
23. Kim YO, Hong SJ, Yim SV. The efficacy of shikonin on cartilage protection in a mouse model of rheumatoid arthritis. Korean J Physiol Pharmacol. 2010;14(4):199–204. (PubMed PMID: 20827333. Pubmed Central PMCID: 2933435).
24. Lee CC, Wang CN, Lai YT, Kang JJ, Liao JW, Chiang BL, et al. Shikonin inhibits maturation of bone marrow-derived dendritic cells and suppresses allergic airway inflammation in a murine model of asthma. Br J Pharmacol. 2010;161(7):1496–511. (PubMed PMID: 20735407. Pubmed Central PMCID: 3010563).
25. Wang XC, Feng J, Huang F, Fan YS, Wang YY, Cao LY, et al. Effects of shikonin isolated from zicao on lupus nephritis in NZB/W F1 mice. Biol Pharm Bull. 2009;32(9):1565–70. (PubMed PMID: 19721233).
26. Xiong J, Ni J, Hu G, Shen J, Zhao Y, Yang L, et al. Shikonin ameliorates cerulein-induced acute pancreatitis in mice. J Ethnopharmacol. 2013;145(2):573–80. (PubMed PMID: 23201088).
27. Singh B, Sharma MK, Meghwal PR, Sahu PM, Singh S. Anti-inflammatory activity of shikonin derivatives from *Arnebia hispidissima*. Phytomedicine. 2003;10(5):375–80. (PubMed PMID: 12834001).
28. Chen X, Oppenheim J, Howard OM. Shikonin, a component of antiinflammatory Chinese herbal medicine, selectively blocks chemokine binding to CC chemokine receptor-1. Int Immunopharmacol. 2001;1(2):229–36. (PubMed PMID: 11360924).
29. Zhang W, Lu QX, Yuan HN. Effect of calculus bovis on immune functions in mice. Zhongguo Zhong Yao Za Zhi. 1993;18(5):302–20. (PubMed PMID: 8216808).
30. Chen X, Mellon RD, Yang L, Dong H, Oppenheim JJ, Howard OM. Regulatory effects of deoxycholic acid, a component of the anti-inflammatory traditional Chinese medicine Niuhuang, on human leukocyte response to chemoattractants. Biochem Pharmacol. 2002;63 (3):533–41. (PubMed PMID: 11853704).
31. Chen X, Yang D, Shen W, Dong HF, Wang JM, Oppenheim JJ, et al. Characterization of chenodeoxycholic acid as an endogenous antagonist of the G-coupled formyl peptide receptors. Inflamm Res. 2000;49(12):744–55. (PubMed PMID: 11211928.).
32. O'Hara R, Murphy EP, Whitehead AS, FitzGerald O, Bresnihan B. Local expression of the serum amyloid A and formyl peptide receptor-like 1 genes in synovial tissue is associated with matrix metalloproteinase production in patients with inflammatory arthritis. Arthritis Rheum. 2004;50(6):1788–99. (PubMed PMID: 15188355).
33. Broughton G. 2nd. Chenodeoxycholate: the bile acid. The drug. a review. Am J Med Sci. 1994;307(1):54–63. (PubMed PMID: 8291509).

34. Palazzi C, D'Amico E, Pennese E, Petricca A. Normalization of methotrexate-induced high levels of serum transaminases after ursodeoxycholic acid administration in a rheumatoid arthritis patient. Rheumatology (Oxford). 2003;42(10):1266–7. (PubMed PMID: 14508047).
35. Bruusgaard A, Andersen RB. Effect of an intravenously administered bile acid (chenodeoxycholic acid) on rheumatoid arthritis. Scand J Rheumatol. 1975;4(3):169–73. (PubMed PMID: 1166284).
36. Chen X, Beutler JA, McCloud TG, Loehfelm A, Yang L, Dong HF, et al. Tannic acid is an inhibitor of CXCL12 (SDF-1alpha)/CXCR4 with antiangiogenic activity. Clin Cancer Res. 2003;9(8):3115–23. (PubMed PMID: 12912963).
37. Buckley CD, Amft N, Bradfield PF, Pilling D, Ross E, Arenzana-Seisdedos F, et al. Persistent induction of the chemokine receptor CXCR4 by TGF-beta 1 on synovial T cells contributes to their accumulation within the rheumatoid synovium. J Immunol. 2000;165(6):3423–9. (PubMed PMID: 10975862).
38. Nanki T, Hayashida K, El-Gabalawy HS, Suson S, Shi K, Girschick HJ, et al. Stromal cell-derived factor-1-CXC chemokine receptor 4 interactions play a central role in CD4+ T cell accumulation in rheumatoid arthritis synovium. J Immunol. 2000;165(11):6590–8. (PubMed PMID: 11086103).
39. Tamamura H, Fujisawa M, Hiramatsu K, Mizumoto M, Nakashima H, Yamamoto N, et al. Identification of a CXCR4 antagonist, a T140 analog, as an anti-rheumatoid arthritis agent. FEBS Lett. 2004;569(1–3):99–104. (PubMed PMID: 15225616).
40. Matthys P, Hatse S, Vermeire K, Wuyts A, Bridger G, Henson GW, et al. AMD3100, a potent and specific antagonist of the stromal cell-derived factor-1 chemokine receptor CXCR4, inhibits autoimmune joint inflammation in IFN-gamma receptor-deficient mice. J Immunol. 2001;167(8):4686–92. (PubMed PMID: 11591799).
41. Mota ML, Thomas G. Barbosa Filho JM. Anti-inflammatory actions of tannins isolated from the bark of Anacardium occidentale L. J Ethnopharmacol. 1985;13(3):289–300. (PubMed PMID: 2414605).
42. Taub DD, Schaffer E. Biological responses to chemokine superfamily members. Curr Protoc Immunol. 2001;Chapter 6:Unit 6 12. (PubMed PMID: 18432804).
43. Pitchford S, Hirst M, Wada HG, Chan SD, Timmermans VE, Humphries GM. Characterization of functional activity of chemokine receptors using the Cytosensor Microphysiometer. Methods Enzymol. 1997;288:84 108. (PubMed PMID: 9356989).
44. June CH. Analysis of lymphocyte activation and metabolism by flow cytometry. Curr Opin Immunol. 1992;4(2):200–4. (PubMed PMID: 1605909).
45. Baly D, Gibson U, Allison D, DeForge L. Biological assays for C-X-C chemokines. Methods Enzymol. 1997;287:69–88. (PubMed PMID: 9330316).
46. Su SB, Gong W, Gao JL, Shen W, Murphy PM, Oppenheim JJ, et al. A seven-transmembrane, G protein-coupled receptor, FPRL1, mediates the chemotactic activity of serum amyloid A for human phagocytic cells. J Exp Med. 1999;189(2):395–402. (PubMed PMID: 9892621. Pubmed Central PMCID: 2192984).
47. Hatse S, Princen K, Liekens S, Vermeire K, De Clercq E, Schols D. Fluorescent CXCL12AF647 as a novel probe for nonradioactive CXCL12/CXCR4 cellular interaction studies. Cytometry A. 2004;61(2):178–88.
48. Zwier JM, Roux T, Cottet M, Durroux T, Douzon S, Bdioui S, et al. A fluorescent ligand-binding alternative using Tag-lite(R) technology. J Biomol Screen. 2010;15(10):1248–59. (PubMed PMID: 20974902).
49. Fukunaga A, Nagai H, Noguchi T, Okazawa H, Matozaki T, Yu X, et al. Src homology 2 domain-containing protein tyrosine phosphatase substrate 1 regulates the migration of Langerhans cells from the epidermis to draining lymph nodes. J Immunol. 2004;172(7):4091–9. (PubMed PMID: 15034021).
50. Chen X, Murakami T, Oppenheim JJ, Howard OM. Triptolide, a constituent of immunosuppressive Chinese herbal medicine, is a potent suppressor of dendritic-cell maturation and trafficking. Blood. 2005;106(7):2409–16. (PubMed PMID: 15956285. Pubmed Central PMCID: 1569904).

MIX
Papier aus verantwortungsvollen Quellen
Paper from responsible sources
FSC® C105338

If you have any concerns about our products,
you can contact us on
ProductSafety@springernature.com

In case Publisher is established outside the EU,
the EU authorized representative is:
Springer Nature Customer Service Center GmbH
Europaplatz 3, 69115 Heidelberg, Germany

Printed by Libri Plureos GmbH
in Hamburg, Germany